HANDBOOK
of SHEN

THE NEW ENERGY/BODY THERAPY
Now Being Used In
HOSPITALS, PAIN CLINICS
ALCOHOL/DRUG TREATMENT CENTERS
AND MENTAL HEALTH FACILITIES

by Richard Rainbow Pavek

This manual is intended for the training of health professionals. Unless you are properly licensed in your state or country, using the procedures described to treat the ailments and disorders discussed may be illegal. (Of course, SHEN may be given to anyone and by anyone for purposes of relaxation and for home and family care.)

Nothing in this manual is intended to imply that all complaints similar to the ones discussed will respond to SHEN procedures nor should the diagnosis of similar appearing disorders be made on the basis of the cases presented.

Neither ownership of this book nor the learning of the techniques described herein entitles one to call themselves a Certified SHEN™ Therapist. Certification is only through approved schools.

ISBN 0-9618646-0-5

Published by THE SHEN THERAPY INSTITUTE at:
No. 20 YFH Gate Six Road, Sausalito, California 94965
415/332-2593

™ SHEN, SHEN Therapy and SHEN Physioemotional Release Therapy are trademarks of the SHEN THERAPY INSTITUTE.

This book is affectionately dedicated to Jane Dohmen whose participation in SHEN, first as a patient, then as investigator and colleague, was more than matched by her encouragement and support through the many years of research.

. . . R.R.P.

PREFACE

Nine and a half years ago I found myself in a loosely styled workshop on "subtle energies" (whatever that meant I did not know). At one point we were instructed to "run energy" through a partner and see if we could balance the temperature in the different parts of their body. I was chosen by a woman whom I did not know and proceeded. I didn't expect much to happen, but shortly after I had placed my hands across her abdomen she began sobbing as her pelvis went into contractions. At the same time, my arms and hands got extremely hot as sweat broke out on my forehead and the hair on my arms began to stand up. The heat and the sobbing increased until they peaked and subsided. When the episode ended, the woman said, "I feel like I just gave birth to myself". Over the next few days it became clear that, while she certainly hadn't given birth to herself, something about her had changed. An emotional weight seemed to have lifted and life seemed different to her. Her new emotional posture maintained over the next several months at which time I lost touch with her.

There was just one problem - for me at least. I simply had not believed that laying on of the hands was anything more than placebo, something occurring mentally to cause internal change. But here was a case where neither of the participants believed anything like this would happen and yet it had. Neither could I deny what I felt in my hands and arms. I was faced with a choice, either expand on my beliefs or check into a psych ward. Given the cost of psych wards, I opted for the former.

I decided to investigate the phenomena but I didn't intend to abandon what I previously knew of science. Since most of my background and training had been in chemistry, electronics and aeronautics, I tended to view the phenomenon as having something to do with fields in physics rather than something in metaphysics or magic. (As to whether or not it was *Spiritual*, this was not an issue for me since I believe that all of everything is spiritual; it was not necessary for me to differentiate.)

After some thought, I decided that it was likely that the field, if indeed it was such, would have to follow the principles of apparent motion that apply to all other field systems in physics, such as magnetism and the formative currents of weather systems. And if this were true, it would mean that once the system was understood, the phenomenon that had occurred could be codified and repeated. Nine and a half years ago I started out to prove this, one way or the other. SHEN is the result.

While SHEN is a new development and does not derive from older methods, there are several medically oriented antecedents. Notable among these is *Polarity Therapy*, which was developed early in this century by Randolph Stone, MD, and *Therapeutic Touch*, developed more recently by Dolores Kreiger, PhD, RN. While there are major differences between SHEN and these two disciplines in theory, approach and application all rely, for the most part, on utilization of the human energy field.

Before that, there was a long history of attempts to utilize "energy" fields in healing. There is documented evidence of this beginning in early Egypt, in China and in India and extending on to the work of Dr. Franz Mesmer in France in the eighteenth century.

While a definitive history of this early work is well beyond the scope of this book (there is more than enough to be covered in theory and practical application) it is fascinating to see how frequently rudimentary methods of using the field in healing physical disorders were discovered, used briefly and then lost, only to be discovered again. And always with a wealth of detractors insisting that if you can't see it or measure it, it must not be real. It is true that the sensory effects noted with the hands are subtle, but the therapeutic results are not. One could say the same about the surgeon's scalpel or about the tiniest drop of curare.

In the past, most attempts to validate the existence of the field and its use in healing physical disorders relied on rather vague metaphysical concepts - statements such as "The physical follows the spiritual", or "The emotional affects the physical". These are true statements, to be sure, and would probably not be questioned by very many. Unfortunately though, casual ideas about the importance of the spiritual and emotional part of the human creature are not much use in a clinical setting. There is no clue in these statements to tell us precisely how one might affect the other nor how one could be manipulated to enhance the other. Whatever results have been obtained by applying these vague "theories" in hands-on practice were not easy to replicate and definately were not explainable within the perspective of the currently accepted medical or psychological models. And certainly not within the physics model. And, it is quite clear that if a field does exist and if it does affect the biophysical body, it must be explainable within these reference frames.

The theoretical foundation for SHEN rests solidly on three interlocking legs, the disciplines of physics, biology and psychology. The theories that have come out of the years of research find logical causes for the effects within current wisdom in these fields. The experiments detailed in Chapter Eight offer compelling evidence that the field does exist, that it is not imaginary.

This book is divided into sections on Theory, Training and Practical Application. (Since this book is intended to be a self-teaching training manual, self review questions appear at several places in the text.)

If your interest is in learning to do SHEN, I suggest that you take the time to read the theoretical portion first, before plunging into the training and application sections. You will find that there is a great deal of material on physiology, biology and psychology that is not found in the usual texts. Most of this is foundational to SHEN and in understanding how to use it effectively in the treatment of difficult disorders.

Over nine years of careful, systematic research has shown, beyond little doubt, that there is a Physioemotional Field that permeates the human body and that this field is involved in the creation and experience of emotion as well as in the formation of tension in the body. It is this double nexus that makes the field the linking mechanism in psychosomatic and somatoform disorders, and the hope for their treatment.

. . . R.R.P. April 17, 1987
Sausalito, California

ACKNOWLEDGEMENTS

A great many people who have encouraged, helped and assisted me in many, many ways over the years in developing SHEN. There is no way that I could thank them all, but a few stand out because of their generous contributions. Among these are: Marlene Baar, MA, Cynthia Beaudry, BSW, Roberta Bodine, RN, Duard Bok, MD, John Bolander, MD, Ursula Campbell, BA, Virginia Connell, MS RN, Elizabeth Crisler, MS RN, Michelle Green, Debra Harris, MD, Sandra Heisler, LVN, Joy Mead-Byrne, MS, Shirley Molenich, MD, Charlotte McClure, MEd, LPC, Lyn McCue, William Newmeyer, MD, John V. Nicholas, PhD. JoAn Owens, Ernest Pecci, MD, Jai Powell, Martin Rossman, MD, Richard Russell, Norman Schwartz, MD, Jean Scott, Jan Sultan, Charles Tart, PhD, Pamela Vantress, Christina Voss, MS, Donald Wilhelm, PhD, David Worthen, CSW and especially the staffs of the: Pain Program, St. Joseph's Hospital, Fort Worth, Texas; Wards 43A & B and 53E & F of the Milwaukee County Mental Health Complex and the Spinal and Chronic Pain Centre, Medical Arts Hospital, Dallas, Texas.

A special debt is owed two men, Frank Lawlis, PhD and Michael Beal, MD for their major assistance in the research undertaken.

Doctor Lawlis's invitation for me to do SHEN in the Pain Clinics he co-heads in Texas became the means to validate and study many of the effects of SHEN and to develop a number of the treatment protocols.

Doctor Beal's invitation to work in Milwaukee and his arranging for research studies on SHEN and Major Depression, and on SHEN and Migraine have been invaluable in the development and validation of the SHEN Procedures. The information gained has taught us much about the range of disorders that can be benefited by SHEN. His thoughtful, patient efforts to guide me in the proper science of systematic research have been most helpful, as has his continuing encouragement, support and friendship.

I also wish to thank Lisa McCann and Jai Powell for their editorial assistance and Natasha Taylor for her illustrations.

To those inadvertently omitted, my apologies.   . . . R.R.P.

CONTENTS

PREFACE _____ v
CONTENTS_____ ix
ILLUSTRATIONS _____ xiii
CASE HISTORIES _____ xiv
TREATMENT PROTOCOLS _____ xiv

CHAPTER 1   INTRODUCTION _____ 1

SECTION I
THE CONNECTION BETWEEN EMOTION AND BIOPHYSICAL DYSFUNCTION
Page 3

CHAPTER 2   THE PHYSIOEMOTIONAL LINK IN EMOTIONALLY ROOTED DISORDERS _____ 5
          Neural Body/Brain Links, 5.   Emotional Body/Brain Links, 6.   Somatic Affect, 6.   Biological Reaction to
          Emotion, 7.   Contractility, 7.   Contraction Around Painful Somatic Affect, 8.   Formation of Long Term
          Disorders, 10.   Regional Stress Effects, 10.   Tables of Emotion Regions, 12.

CHAPTER 3   RESULTS OF RELEASING PHYSIOEMOTIONAL CONTRACTILE TENSIONS
              IN TWENTY-FIVE SHEN CASES _____ 13
          Interventions at the Lower Gastrointestinal Region, 15.
          Interventions at the Umbilical Region, 17.
          Interventions at the Umbilicus/Pubic/Iliac Region, 20.
          Interventions at the Epigastric/Hypochondriac Region, 22.
          Interventions at the Heart Region, 24.
          Interventions at the Perineum Region, 27.

          Review of Chapters 2 and 3, 30.

CHAPTER 4   BIOLOGICAL CONSEQUENCES OF CONTRACTION _____ 31
          Capillary Perfusion, 31.   Organic Factors in Tension, 32.

CHAPTER 5   APPROACHES TO DYSFUNCTION
              PSYCHOSOMATIC VERSUS INVOLUNTARY CONTRACTION _____ 33
          The Psychosomatic Concept, 33.   The Concept of Contractility, 33.   The Patient and Contractility, 33.
          Psychosomatic Brain/Body Pathways, 34.   Involuntary Brain/Body Pathways, 35.

          Review of Chapters 4 and 5, 36.

SECTION II
EMOTION AND PHYSICS
Page 37

CHAPTER 6   EMOTION AND PHYSICS _____ 39
          The Two Basic Effects of Emotion, 40.   Body Movement in Relation to Emotion, 40.   Perception of Somatic
          Location of Emotion, 41.   Differing Stress Results of Different Emotions, 42.   Composition of Emotion -
          Biochemical? or Something Else?, 42.

          Review of Chapter 6, 44.

CHAPTER 7   **FIELD-LIKE EFFECTS OF EMOTION** _____ *45*

Feeling Emotions of Others, 45.   Pheromones, 46.   The Mental Model of Emotion, 47.   Differences between Thoughts and Emotions, 47.   Rational Thought, 49.   Confusion? or Confused Thought?, 50. Biochemical Model of Emotion, 51.   The Fight or Flight Response, 52.   Examining the Experience of Fear, 53.   The Energy Field Model of Fight or Flight, 54.   Which Came First? Emotion or Biochemical Change, 54. The Field Theory of Emotion, 55.

Review of Chapter 7, 56.

CHAPTER 8   **PHYSICS OF THE PHYSIOEMOTIONAL FIELD** _____ *57*

The Question of Evidence, 57.   Establishing the Nature of the Field, 58.   Other Experiments, 59. Organization and Pattern of the Flows, 61.   The Three Part Pattern, 64.   Field Action at the Emotion Centers, 66.   Some Difficult Questions, 70.

Review of Chapter 8, 72.

SECTION III
LEARNING TO DO SHEN
Page 73

CHAPTER 9   **BASIC SHEN** _____ *75*

Learning to Sense the Field, 75.   Determining the Direction of your Arm/Hand Flow, 76. General Instructions for Doing SHEN Flows, 78.   First Practice Session (Day 1), 80.   Second Practice Session (Day 1), 82.

Review Questions for Chapter 9, 84.

First Outside Practice Session, 85.
Second Outside Practice Session, 86.

CHAPTER 10   **SHEN FLOWS AT THE EMOTION CENTERS** _____ *87*

Definitions, 87.   Working With the Emotion Regions, 88.   Shoulder/Head Flows, 90.   First Practice Session (Day 2), 91.   Notations, 92.   Second Practice Session (Day 2), 93.   Transverse Flows, 93.   Crown Flows, 94.   Third Practice Session (Day 2), 94.

Third Outside Practice Session (Solar Plexus) 95.
Fourth Outside Practice Session (Heart) 96.
Fifth Outside Practice Session (Pubic) 97.
Sixth Outside Practice Session (Throat and Root) 98.

CHAPTER 11   **ADVANCED SHEN PROCEDURES** _____ *99*

Expanded Root and Crown Flows, 99.   Frontal Flows, 100.   First Practice Session (Day 3), 101.   Flows at the Sides, 102.   Combining Flows Through Two Centers, 103.   Second Practice Session (Day 3), 105. Points to Remember, 105.

Review of Chapter 10 and 11, 106.

SECTION IV
CLINICAL AND THERAPEUTIC SHEN
Page 107

CHAPTER 12   **SHEN SELF FLOWS** _____ *109*
     Doing SHEN on Yourself, 109.

CHAPTER 13   **PLANNING THE SESSION AND DEVELOPING THE TREATMENT SERIES** _____ *111*
     Planning the Session, 111. Developing the Treatment Series, 112. Scheduling, 112. Some Rules of Thumb, 113. Instructions to give the client, 114

CHAPTER 14   **COMBINING SHEN AND OTHER THERAPIES** _____ *115*
     Breathwork, Rebirthing, 115. Massage, 115. Imagery, 115. Gestalt, 116. Rolfing, 116.

CHAPTER 15   **SHEN THERAPY FOR EMOTIONAL AND PSYCHIATRIC DISORDERS** _____ *117*
     Major Depression, 117. Fear of Insanity, 118. Phobias, Anxiety Attacks, Patient in crisis, 118. Recurrent Images, Dreams, Nightmares, 119. Hallucinations, 119. General Considerations, 120. Children's Night Terrors, 121. Patient Management, 121.

CHAPTER 16   **EFFECTS OF SHEN ON THE "KUNDILINI CRISIS"** _____ *123*
     Pain During Meditation, 123. Ecstasy Turning to Pain, 124. Falling Out, 124. Kriyas, 125. Siddhas, 126.

CHAPTER 17   **SHEN IN THE HOSPITAL AND CLINIC** _____ *127*
     Panacea or Specific, 127. Swollen Tissue, 127. Pain, 127. Improving Organ Function, 128. Emotionally Influenced Disorders, 128. Physical Disorders with Emotional Results, 128. Emotionally Rooted Disorders, 128. SHEN in the Hospital, 129. Pre & Post Surgery Procedures, 130. Psychogenic Shock, Some Coma, 131. Fractures, Swollen and Sprained Joints, 131. Arthritis, 131. Bursitis, 131. Kidney Stones, 132. Gallstones, 132. Aches and Pains of the Aged, 132. Muscle Tension Headaches, 132. Sinus Headaches, 132. Pregnancy and Birthing, 133. Vertigo, Tinnitus, 133. Jet Lag, 133. Protocols for Emotionally Rooted Disorders, 134. Irritable Bowel Syndrome, 134. Migraine and Migraine Variants, 135. Premenstrual and Menstrual Distress, 137. Anorexia/Eating Disorders, 138.

CHAPTER 18   **SHEN AND CHRONIC PAIN** _____ *139*
     Psychological Responses to Pain, 139. Major Pain Components in Chronic Pain Syndrome, 139. Development of Simple Chronic Pain, 140. Pre Injury Fear, 140. Post Injury Fear, 141. Non-Injury Related Emotional Components, 141. Emergence of Memory, 142. Development of Complex Chronic Pain, 142. Psychogenic Pain, 142. Chronic Low Back Syndrome, 144. Unremitting Psychogenic Pain Stemming From a Strong Blow, 145. Determining the Degree of Psychogenisity, 145. Expectations With Various Patients, 145. Patient Management and Concerns, 146.

SECTION V

APPENDIX A   **CASE HISTORY** _____ *149*

APPENDIX B   **THE SHEN NOTATION SYSTEM** _____ *163*

BIBLIOGRAPHY _____ *165*

INDEX _____ *167*

ILLUSTRATIONS

Figure		Page
1	The Amoeba	7
2	Somatic Effects of Some Repressed Emotions	29
3	Psychosomatic Brain/Body Pathways	34
4	Involuntary Brain/Body Pathways	35
5	Field Effects	49
6	Temperature Measurement	58
7	Temperature Measurements Through Insulation	58
8	Recording the Flow	59
9	Flows at Successive Sites	60
10	Normal Flow	60
11	Reversed Flow	61
12	Peripheral Flows	62
13	Magnetic Field Connections	62
14	Peripheral Flow Connections	62
15	The Halo Effect	62
16	Spinal Flow	62
17	Magnet and Arm Flows	63
18	Increasing the Flows	63
19	Peripheral, Arm and Spinal Flows	63
20	Formation of Clouds	64
21	Passing Under a Cloud	64
22	Complete Patterns in Fields	65
23	Field Around the Arms	65
24	Matching the Helices	65
25	The Body Helices	65
26	The Centers of Emotion	66
27	Sound Waves	67
28	Rotating the Bubble	67
29	Forming the Vortices	67
30	Compressed Centers	68
31	Return Flows	68
32	Blocking Segments	68
33	Emotion Regions	69
34	Crossing Fields	70
35	Mixing the Flows	70
36	The Combined Flows	70
37	Transformer Action	71
38	Breath and the "Pump"	71
39	Sensing the Field	75
40	Rotating the Hands	75
41	Determining Flow Direction	76
42	Suggestion or Real?	77
43	Hot Spot	78
44	Direction of Flow	79
45	Merging Flows	79
46	Shorting Out	79
47	Peripheral and Arm Flows	80

Figure		Page
48	Overlapping the Segments	80
49	Head Loop	81
50	Arm, Spine & Peripherals	82
51	Emotion Center Flows	83
52	Root Flows	83
53	Arm, Spine & Peripherals	85
54	Head Loop	85
55	Root Flows	85
56	Peripheral & Arm Flows	86
57	Emotion Center Flows	86
58	Root Flows	86
59	Some Definitions	87
60	Locating the Centers	87
61	Flow Directions	88
62	Multiple Flows	88
63	Simplified Triples	88
64	Locations of Frontward Triples (Emotion Regions)	89
65	Locations of Rearward Triples (Blocking Segments)	89
66	Shoulder/Head Flows	90
67	Kath Session, First Part	91
68	Kath Session, Second Part	91
69	Precise Locations	92
70	Transverse Flows	93
71	Crown Flows	94
72	Solar Plexus Flows	95
73	Heart Flows	96
74	Pubic Flows	97
75	Throat and Root Flows	98
76	Expanding the Root Flows	99
77	Expanding the Crown Flows	99
78	Frontal Flows	100
79	Right and Wrong Ways	100
80	Working From the Front	100
81	Available Directions	101
82	First Session, Day 3	101
83	SHEN Flows at the Sides	102
84	Diagonals at the Sides	102
85	Similarities Between Root & Frontward Comb. Flows	103
86	Frontward Combinations	103
87	Similarities Between Crown & Rearward Comb. Flows	104
88	Rearward Combinations	104
89	Combination Diagonals	104
90	Second Session Day 3	105
91	BiPhasic Breathing	111
92	Simple Chronic Pain	140
93	Complex Chronic Pain	142
94	To Reverse Force of a Blow	143

CASE HISTORIES

Alcoholism	119
Anorexia	22
Appetite loss after trauma	23
Auditory hallucinations	118
Back pain	17-19, 21, 141-143
Bowel complaints	16
Broken leg	32
Bulimia	22
Chest pains	24
Chronic back pain	17-19, 21, 142, 143
Cluster headache	27
Coma, psychogenic	27
Depression,	
major	118
psychotic	119
Digestive complaints	15
Eating disorders	22, 23
Ecstasy turning to pain	124
Falling out	124
Fear of insanity	118
Gastrointestinal	15, 22
Headaches	25-27
Hypertension	24
Insanity, fear of	118
Irritable bowel syndrome	16
Kriyas	125
Loss of appetite	23
Low back syndrome	17-19, 21
Major depression	118
Meditation, pain during	123
Menstrual	
bleeding, severe	21
distress	20-21
Migraine	25, 26, 149
Night terrors	28
Pain,	
back	141
chronic low back	17-19, 21, 142, 143
during meditation	123
secondary	141
Post traumatic stress disorder	28
Premenstrual distress	20,21
Psychogenic pain	143
Psychogenic shock	27
Psychotic depression	119
Schizophrenia	118
Shock, psychogenic	27
Siddhas	125
Spastic colon	16
Swollen leg	32

TREATMENT PROTOCOLS

Abdominal migraine	135
Acephalgia	135
Aches & pains of the aged	132
Anorexia	138
Appetite loss	130
Arthritis	131
Back pain	144
Birthing	133
Blow, pain from a	143
Broken bones	131
Bulimia	138
Bursitis	131
Children's night terrors	121
Chronic pain,	
low back	144
from a blow	143
Coma, psychogenic	131
Crohn's disease	138
Cyclical vomiting	135
Eating disorders	138
Fractures	131
Gallstones, 132	
Gastroenteritis	138
Headaches,	
migraine	135-136
other	132
Hydrocephalus	133
Irritable bowel syndrome	134
Jet lag	133
Kidney stones	131
Low back pain	144
Menstrual	
bleeding, excessive	137
distress	137
Migraine and variants	135-136
Night terrors, children's	121
Pain, from blow	143
Pregnancy	133
Premenstrual distress	137
Psychosomatic disorders	134
Shock, psychogenic	131
Sinus headaches	132
Spastic colon	134
Sprains	131
Stones,	
gall,	132
kidney	132
Surgery, support of	130
Swollen joints	131
Tension headaches	132
Tinnitus	133
Vertigo	133

CHAPTER 1

INTRODUCTION

SHEN (Specific Human Energy Nexus) Physioemotional Release Therapy™ is a series of non-invasive touch relaxation procedures that are beginning to be used in hospitals, behavioral medicine and chronic pain clinics for the relief of a number of emotionally rooted disorders including psychogenic chronic pain, premenstrual and menstrual distress, migraine and cluster headache, psychogenic shock and some eating disorders and heart pain. Because of its ability to release deeply repressed emotion, SHEN also has application in the treatment of a range of troublesome stress-linked and emotion-related disorders including depression, anxiety and the phobias, as well as assisting the client in crisis.

When the pressureless touch procedures comprising SHEN are applied to the body, the involuntary physioemotional tensions that surround the sites of either physical pain or emotional pain are released. When these tensions are dissolved, their effect on the local body region inside them also ends, and the glands and organs in that region become free to function normally. When these tensions cease, quite dramatic reductions in chronic pain and the other primary symptoms often occur. And they occur rapidly.

The vehicle that the SHEN Therapist uses to achieve these results is the portion of the physioemotional field (also called the biofield or energy field), that extends between the therapist's hands. This field permeates all human bodies, making it possible for one person to effect another's field and cause beneficial change.

But is there really such a thing as a "field of energy" in and around the human body? No doubt some who have read this far do not accept the existence of this field. To convince yourself that it does exist, turn now to Chapter Nine, page 75 and do the simple tests that allow you to sense it for yourself. Perhaps not everyone will be able to detect the field immediately, but those who do will be able to read the theory presented in this book with something more than blind faith. *You may also wish to read of the laboratory experiments that are detailed in Chapter Eight, pages 58-61.*

There is no single theory that explains the nature of the physioemotional field nor its effects on the physical body and its relationship to emotion. There are three interlocking theories. One relates how somatic emotion, the bodily experience of the emotions, can manifest as psychosomatic and somatoform disorders when repressed. Another describes laws of motion in physics that govern emotional effects between people while the third covers the effects of tension on biological dysfunction.

At first glance the theoretical footings of SHEN sound somewhat ridiculous: after all, what could physics have to do with emotion? And what is this nonsense about emotion appearing in the body?

I think when you read the theories, you will find that the assemblage of facts presented offers interesting answers for a number of perplexing questions, including the big one of

---

™ SHEN, SHEN Therapy and SHEN Physioemotional Release Therapy are trade marks of the SHEN THERAPY INSTITUTE, Sausalito, California.

how it is possible for emotion to translate into biophysical dsyfunction. Beyond that, these theories do not violate current wisdom in biology, psychology and physics. The theories expand on those disciplines, not negate them. You will find that you need take no "leaps of faith" nor will you have to make any more of an effort to keep an open mind than you have so far.

* * * * *

As to the effects achieved with SHEN Therapy, there are many who have tried to say that it is just placebo, that it is all psychological, all in the mind. I do not believe that this is true as there is just too much evidence supportive of SHEN's effectiveness. Placebos simply do not have a success rate of over sixty percent. SHEN does, with all disorders where it is indicated. But, even if it were placebo, it would seem to me that a placebo which ends most migraines in the middle of an attack without the support of any medication, one that can radically improve premenstrual distress symptoms and can end many cases of chronic low back pain, would be worth investigating. (As to whether it is a placebo or not, it is interesting to note that the precise SHEN procedures that are effective with one disorder will not help another disorder that is aided by a different procedure. This is more like the actions of specifics than like those of placebos.)

Not all cases attempted are successful, to be sure, but a high percentage are, far higher than from one that is just a benign placebo. Single blind studies on the effects of SHEN with several disorders are underway. (Double blind studies are out of the question, of course.) The model of attainable health and well-being that is emerging from these theories is being amply validated by the results of the various SHEN treatment protocols.

* * * * *

Learning to use SHEN effectively is not at all difficult, as you will discover when you practice the techniques in this book, and requires no special abilities nor any particular philosophical orientation or spiritual belief. Nor is it necessary to be particularly intuitive or psychic. (If you are, so much the better, after you learn SHEN you will know how to use that information effectively.) The techniques, as with other methods based on science, require thoughtful, attentive and intelligent application.

You will find that the investment of time is more than worth the effort. Once you have learned the SHEN techniques, you will be able to successfully treat a number of previously perplexing disorders, disorders that have defied previous methods. And you will be able to bring relief to many who have given up hope.

> NOTE: Because there are many technical terms used in the
> health professional field that are not precisely interchangeable
> between the divisions of the field, I have defined these terms
> wherever it seemed necessary.

SECTION I
THE CONNECTION BETWEEN EMOTION AND BIOPHYSICAL DYSFUNCTION
Page 3

*Stress is always taken to be a systemic condition. We have considered the results of any and all stressful emotions to be systemic, even as we have been aware of their localized effects. As long as we continue to use the single word, **stress**, to cover the results of all emotions in the body, we will never see that each emotion is an individual stressor, each having specific results in local body regions.*

CHAPTER 2   **THE PHYSIOEMOTIONAL LINK IN EMOTIONALLY ROOTED DISORDERS**   *5*
Neural Body/Brain Links, 5.   Emotional Body/Brain Links, 6.   Somatic Affect, 6.   Biological Reaction to Emotion, 7.   Contractility, 7.   Contraction Around Painful Somatic Affect, 8.   Formation of Long Term Disorders, 10.   Regional Stress Effects, 10.   Tables of Emotion Regions, 12.

CHAPTER 3   **RESULTS OF RELEASING PHYSIOEMOTIONAL CONTRACTILE TENSIONS IN TWENTY-FIVE SHEN CASES**   *13*
Interventions at the Lower Gastrointestinal Region, 15.
Interventions at the Umbilical Region, 17.
Interventions at the Umbilicus/Pubic/Iliac Region, 20.
Interventions at the Epigastric/Hypochondriac Region, 22.
Interventions at the Heart Region, 24.
Interventions at the Perineum Region, 27.

Review of Chapters 2 and 3, 30.

CHAPTER 4   **BIOLOGICAL CONSEQUENCES OF CONTRACTION**   *31*
Capillary Perfusion, 31.   Organic Factors in Tension, 32.

CHAPTER 5   **APPROACHES TO DYSFUNCTION**
PSYCHOSOMATIC VERSUS INVOLUNTARY CONTRACTION   *33*
The Psychosomatic Concept, 33.   The Concept of Contractility, 33.   The Patient and Contractility, 33. Psychosomatic Brain/Body Pathways, 34.   Involuntary Brain/Body Pathways, 35.

Review of Chapters 4 and 5, 36.

That the emotional state affects the physical is largely unquestioned, but just how it does that has remained veiled. Even more so is just *how* the specific thoughts generated in a particular psychosocial situation might precipitate a long term physical disorder and why one person's body would respond so differently from another person's, when both were affected by identical emotionally charged incidents.

CHAPTER 2

THE PHYSIOEMOTIONAL LINK
IN
EMOTIONALLY ROOTED DISORDERS

For years, psychological factors have been implicated as being causal in a number of biophysical disorders. Indeed, at one time or another, the medical texts have referenced quite a range of disorders as stemming from these causative factors. These disorders have several common threads. Usually they are nuisance disorders, generally untreatable, bothersome to the physician, draining the physician's and nurse's time. The list includes everything from chronic low back pain, irritable bowel syndrome, premenstrual syndrome, migraine, heart disorders, to ulcers, the list goes on and on. It must be said, however, that as the range of drugs available to treat the *symptoms* of these disorders has broadened and "cures" effected, the list has been shortened. The implication is; if it can be cured by a drug or a vitamin it must not have been psychological in origin. Never mind that the psychological factors and emotional derivatives linked with the disorders have not changed - a cap has been put on the most noticeable physical aspects of the disorder and it can be set aside. Never mind if the patient is relegated to a lifetime of drug taking. This may be good medicine but is it good healing? To some, at least, the patient is more than just a biological body.

It may well be that the proliferation of symptom masking medicines has blinded us to the real underlying causes. It is well accepted that many drugs do nothing more than mask pain and other biological or physiological symptoms. It is also well known that many drugs alter the overt emotional state without affecting the psychological or mental state. Why should we think that drugs which offset the grosser symptoms in dysfunctions such as premenstrual syndrome, spastic colon and other emotionally rooted disorders are doing anything more than masking the real basis of the disorder?

Not everyone agrees with the premise that drugs cure these disorders. Those disagreeing include the many psychologists who feel they are on the edge of grasping the nature of the problem, a great many doctors and nurses who know they are merely providing a stop gap to the problem but have nothing else to offer and a large, very large, group of increasingly dissatisfied patients, who view long term drugs as crutches and who want to get well.

THE NEURAL BODY/BRAIN LINK
The certainty of the psychogenic or psychoplastic[1] effects of psychological factors has been obscured by the lack of clearly defined pathways between the brain and the rest of the physical body. Because it links the brain and the body in most life functions, the neurological system has been the chief focus, in fact almost the only focus, of the search. But because its effects are so pervasive and universal to the entire body, it has been

---

[1] The term **psychogenic** means causing pathology and the term **psychoplastic** means shaping pathology.

virtually impossible to sort out its specific part, if any, in the mind-body connections in specific psychosomatic and somatoform[2] disorders.

Certainly neurological factors are involved, but the way in which they are has not been at all clear. The broad scale introduction of norepinephrine, epinephrine, endorphins and other neurological agents into the total body in the face of stressful situations does not explain why individual disorders spring up in individual people. While we cannot ignore the neurological system, as it must be part of the total mechanism involved, it is becoming obvious that we must look elsewhere for the main organizing principle.

THE EMOTIONAL BRAIN/BODY LINKS

There is another, somewhat neglected, factor that is common to both the mental or psychological aspects and to the physical aspects of these disorders. This factor is *emotion*. Emotions are often dismissed as being merely a subset of the mental process but this subordinating view overlooks the magnitude of the part they play in the body's physiological processes.

Emotions are perhaps the most important activating and determining factor in the state of the physiological body as a whole as well as of its various regions, though how they do this has not been well understood. On reflection though, it is easy to spot a clue - *the sensations of the various emotions pervade the human body*, and they do this at least as much as the nervous system does. Emotions are not only an integral part of the psychological background of every psychosomatic or somatoform disorder; they are experienced in the mind as *thoughts* as well as appearing in the body as *somatic affect*[3]. This dual residency makes emotions a principle linking mechanism between the mind and the body in psychosomatic, somatoform and conversion disorders and a major factor in other disorders as well.

It is generally accepted that the limbic system is involved with the emotional experience in the body. Probably most authorities would hold that the brain furnishes impulses that are spread by the limbic system through the body to cause the experience of somatic affect. However there are other authorities who suggest that it may be the other way around, that the body may be furnishing impulses to the brain. (For the moment we will avoid the argument and focus on what is important to the thrust of this chapter; the existence of an innate, biological reaction of the body to painful somatic affect.)

---

[2] It is generally accepted that psychosomatic disorders are associated with the **suppression** of emotion (stemming from a conscious process) and that somatoform disorders derive from the **repression** of emotion (stemming from an unconscious process). The physiological processes involved appear to be the same, regardless of the difference in attitudenal position, and SHEN procedures would be the same in either case.

[3] Affect means mood or feeling state. a: Somatic Affect is that portion of the total emotional experience which is perceived in the torso. It is the experience of specific bodily sensations and feelings that are associated with a particular emotion. Somatic Affect is differentiated from bodily expression of emotion i.e. facial **expression**, limb and extremity **movement**. b: The Somatic Affects of the different emotions differ considerably from one another. The particular somatic affect of sadness is experienced differently from the somatic affect of anger, or of shame or the other emotions. c: Some Somatic Affects are pleasant and desired (i.e. love, joy) and others are unpleasant and painful (grief, shame, etc.).

THE BIOLOGICAL REACTION TO EMOTION

The connections between a good emotional state and good physical health and between a poor emotional state and poor health are well known, and most would accept that both sets are two way streets - either good health or good emotional state can cause the other with the same being true for poor emotional states and poor physical health. Now the simplicity of these two statements might cause one to jump to the conclusion that there is nothing but a mental *parallel* between good-feeling emotions and good physical health and between bad-feeling emotions and bad physical health; i.e., if you mentally feel good you will be physically healthy and if you feel bad emotionally you will be physically worse off. If we do this we overlook an important, basic difference in the body's physiological reaction to good emotions and to bad emotions.

Essentially the difference is this: *when the emotional state is good the body does not react*, instead it just purrs along healthily, running as is intended. A good emotional state is the norm, or at least should be, and the body has nothing to react to or against. Emotions that are pleasurable, such as love, joy, the feeling of high self esteem do not cause good health, because good health is the norm. However, when faced with bad or painful emotions the body reacts away from its normal, pleasurable state with a specific, definite reaction and can develop a state of poor health.

The body's reaction to painful somatic affect is quite a different process from its non-reaction to pleasurable somatic affect. Pleasurable somatic affects are rarely avoided, nor are the emotionally tinged thoughts that accompany them. We enjoy them and try to perpetuate them. But when emotions occur that we experience as being painful; sadness, fear and shame for example, we not only try to avoid them mentally, the body reacts against the painful somatic affect by automatically contracting around the pain site. (This is the identical reaction the body has to the experience of physical pain.)

It is this innate bodily reaction to the somatic affects of these universally painful emotions that sets the stage for emotionally rooted psychobiological disorders.

CONTRACTILITY: THE AUTOMATIC BIOLOGICAL RESPONSE TO PAIN.

Contractility is an automatic response to pain that is inherent in all living creatures. All life forms, from the amoeba to the human, respond to the intrusion of pain by involuntary contraction. The amoeba, when touched from any quarter, does not move away from the intrusion but withdraws or contracts into itself.

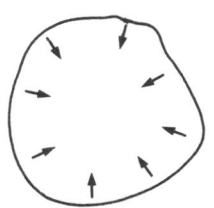

Figure 1
The Amoeba

This contraction develops concentrically around the site of the intrusion. Probably this reaction was necessary for the survival of these early life forms.

Contractile Effect

Since these primitive life forms did not have the ability to discriminate and reason, they could not sense the direction of danger (the pain) nor be able to withdraw from it. Their only defensive maneuver would be to contract, that is, withdraw from all directions at once. Now, it could be argued that since the amoeba has no means of locomotion and must necessarily contract in order to withdraw, and that humans are not so limited, automatic contraction need not occur in human beings. Perhaps not, but the same effect is readily noted in humans and is easy to demonstrate. Just slip up behind someone and poke them in the side and watch how their body pulls into a hunched over posture even before they begin to move away. The action you will see is one of collapsing around the poked site, not one of moving away. This automatic contractile reaction did not disappear during evolution as the need for it changed but remains an inherent human physiological characteristic, one that has unfortunate consequences when activated by painful emotion.

Now the problem occurs because the sensory mechanisms in the periphery of the body do not have the ability to discriminate between external and internal pain. The sensory mechanism that triggers the contraction is much like the action of an electric fence which sounds the alarm if approached and touched from the outside. But electrical fences are directionally blind and will sound the alarm just as rapidly when touched from the inside as they do when touched from the outside.

The body's directional blindness to physical pain is readily observed in the reaction called the *splinting reflex*. When a bone in the body is broken the muscles around the bone automatically contract and apply tension to immobilize it. This response does not extend throughout the entire body, but is focused around the pain of the break as the rest of the muscles are free to move normally. Clearly this reflexive response is neither a learned one nor a conscious one.

Not everyone has had the experience of a broken bone to reference, but most of us have had the experience of sharp intestinal gas pains. Without intending it, we often find that our body has contracted to hold in the pain. Of course it can be argued that this may be a learned response - that sometime in the past we discovered that intentional inward pressure would offset the outward pressure of the gas and neutralize the pain as well as any possible damage. Whether or not it was initially a learned response or was an inherent biological holdover from the amoeba is immaterial. What is important here is that the response now occurs without conscious reasoning.

CONTRACTION AROUND PAINFUL SOMATIC AFFECT

The experience of painful somatic affect appears to trigger the same response that physical pain does. This is because the emotions of sadness, fear, shame for example, generate sensory feeling states, or somatic affect, that the physical body experiences as painful. Those feeling sensations hurt, and the body tries to avoid those hurts.

The examples of painful somatic affect and the body's response to them are legion and have happened to us all. There are few of us who at one time or another have not been aware of how the feeling of sadness pains the heart or how the pain of shame stabs the lower gut. Often these are transient pains that dissolve almost instantly into the next emerging emotion. They may not be so brief however, they may remain to trouble us for a time by hampering our normal response to life. The residue of these painful emotions can, over time, slowly convert into physical dysfunction.

The heart feels a stab of sadness or grief and suddenly it is hard to draw a breath. Often small children filled with sudden sadness have such difficulty drawing a breath that they may have to be coaxed to breathe. And as they do begin to breathe they begin to cry. With older people the stab of grief that is denied physical experience can soon develop into an angina and the angina into more serious heart problems if the grief is not dealt with properly. Some sources indicate that perhaps as many as sixty percent of patients in cardiac units suffered a major grief within six months prior to a heart attack. With most of these patients further investigation reveals that they never completed the physical grieving process. This is not meant to imply that all heart attacks are emotionally caused events. And it is not to say that hardened arteries are not valid predisposing factors. It is more likely that the combination of the two conditions is the culprit, the contraction of the grief compounded the already lessened blood flow caused by the narrowed arteries.

The contraction effect is also seen in the person who is running to avoid an attacker, while desperately trying to breathe. Obviously full breathing is vital to provide for the sudden increased need for oxygen but the person's diaphragm is half paralyzed with fear. What paralyzes it? The center of the somatic experience of fear is the region of the Solar Plexus which is also the location of the diaphragm. As the diaphragm relaxes in order to expand and take in air, the somatic affect of fear begins to emerge. This triggers the contraction which attempts to stop the painful somatic affect. A normal body movement has become painful because of a painful emotion. This programmed response to pain occurs well below the conscious level and is so imbedded in the basic biological structure that it is extremely difficult to deactivate with conscious effort. Anyone who has tried to draw a full breath while filled with fear will attest to the difficulty.

Sometimes the validity of my theories is brought home to me rather forcefully. Recently I was on a white-water rafting expedition and was thrown from the raft when we hit a partially submerged rock. As I was thrown, I grabbed a rope fastened to a tie point on the raft. Somehow my finger caught between the rope and the raft and dislocated as the raft and I went our separate ways. There I was, frightened of drowning because I do not swim well, fearful for my turned around finger, bobbing through the rapids, banging on rocks and desperately trying to breath. And desperately trying to breath was exactly what was happening because every breath took a real, concentrated effort.

Each time I tried to draw a breath the fear increased dramatically and my body tried to stop it by contracting around it. I could actually feel it contract and leave me breathless. Every breath took a major conscious effort to overcome the contraction. Part of my mind did actually recognize the significance of the event as it related to the theory being presented here, but it was a very small part. Most of my mental effort was caught in fighting to overcome the fear response that was keeping my diaphragm contracted.

Similar effects are noted for the other painful somatic affects. One situation where it is often noted is in patients with irritable bowel syndrome. "An emotionally stressful interview may increase colonic contractile activity in certain patients" (Almy 1949). This is an involuntary action, one that the sufferer is usually fighting against.

THE FORMATION OF LONG-TERM DISORDERS

If these contractions were transient there would be little likelihood of their causing long-term dysfunction in the body. A fleeting moment of contraction would be of small concern, it would pass and its effects would pass. The problem begins when emotion is repressed and is never normally experienced. This is because, when and as the contraction eases and the region relaxes, the unresolved painful somatic affect will re-emerge, and re-trigger the contraction. This re-enforcing feedback loop creates constant tension in the region as it traps the pain inside. It is hard to believe that this constant tension would not adversely impact on organ function.

It is through continued suppression of unwanted, painful emotions that the body's organic functions are affected, and it is through the release of these contractile tensions that proper organic function can be restored.[4]

REGIONAL STRESS EFFECTS: *Specific disorders from specific emotions*

If there are systemic effects of emotion, it follows that the results would necessarily be dominated and shaped by the individual's dominant emotional set and would therefore result in different disorders. We all recognize that no two people will have the same emotional response to the same emotional situation. We also recognize that their response will be dictated by their emotional history; by which emotional issues they have resolved or not resolved. Two people faced with an angry employer may respond quite differently - one may burst into tears and the other may flare and then repress anger in response. Considering this, it is no surprise that two individuals present different disorders that seem to be caused by the same trauma. It is not far fetched to imagine that one of these might develop ulcers but not the other. The other would be more likely to develop either chronic low back pain or experience an exacerbation of premenstrual distress. But what are the factors that differentiate between those two people, the factors that determine which one succumbs to which disorder?

The determining factor is in the specific location in the body of the somatic affect being repressed by the contraction . Examination of the contractile effect shows that *the epicenter of contraction is not at the center of body mass,* but changes according to the emotion being experienced. *It is the regional emotional state of the body that determines susceptibility of that region to discord*. The effects of contraction are not spread evenly across the body, but are focused around the particular somatic affect.

The idea of anatomic specificity, that certain disorders tend to group within certain psychological parameters, is not new. Adler (around 1910) suggested the idea of "Organ Inferiority". Franz Alexander and his associates (1950) proposed "Typical Specific Constellations", the idea that certain specific disorders constellate within certain emotional conflict parameters. Other early researchers have proposed a number of organic and psychological approaches including concepts of "Particular Attitudes" (Grace & Graham 1952), "Predisposing Organic States" (Sternbach 1966, Schwartz 1977), and "Individual Response Specificity" (Engel 1960). However, as fruitful as this pioneering work was, it did not produce a key to ending these disorders.

---

[4] It is important to realize that it is not the **experience** of the emotions that causes the disorder but the continued **suppression** of the emotion.

10

Common awareness teaches us that all somatic affect is site specific. The bodily experiences of emotion do not all occur in the same region of the body. There are five principle centers, or regions, where these sensory effects are experienced. These regions are: the *heart, solar plexus, navel, pubic and groin/perineum* (junction of the legs). The emotions associated with each region are different.

For example, the heart region generates the somatic affects associated with the emotions of love, sadness, reverence and grief. Repression of any of these emotions can result in temporary pain and shortness of breath or when repressed more severely for longer terms can lead to angina and grief-related congestive heart failure.

In 1977, Bartrop, et al., published the results of a study that showed lowered **T cell activity** (but not activity of other immune factors) in grieving, surviving spouses. Why T cells and not the other immune factors? Because grief causes contractions around the heart and the thymus, activator of the T cells, resides in the region of the heart.

The relation of body region dysfunction to specific emotion is also illustrated in a recent pilot study designed to test the effects of SHEN Therapy performed at the navel/pubic region on women presenting with premenstrual and menstrual distress. (This region contains both the uterus and the ovaries and is the location where somatic affects of confidence and shame are normally experienced and/or repressed.)

Eleven of the thirteen patients who had SHEN performed during the premenstrual or menstrual phase reported a lowering of symptoms. Twelve reported that emotions of being violated, victimized, embarrassed, sexually aroused, happy, sad, panicked, hysterical, fearful, anxious, depressed, and/or feelings of self abasement, occurred during the session. Five reported that memories of psychically debilitating childhood events surfaced during the SHEN session (some of these memories had not previously been available for recall). Twelve reported a feeling of well being following the treatment.

The correlations between sites of emotion and sites of dysfunction are shown in the tables on the next page.

Table 1   **REGIONS OF SOMATIC AFFECT AND RELATED ORGAN DYSFUNCTION**

Emotion	Somatic Affect at the	Disorder	Presents at the
Love Grief or Sadness	Heart	Congestive Heart Failure following grief Hypertension Angina Pectoris Migraine[5]	Heart Region
Anger Fear Anxiety	Solar Plexus	Anorexia Digestive Disorders Ulcers	Epigastric/ Hypochondriac Region
Guilt,Shame Security Confidence Helplessness	Navel/Pubic	Premenstrual Syndrome Irritable Bowel Syndrome Chronic Low Back Pain	L4/L5/S1 & Ovaries
Mortal Fear	Groin/Perineum	Psychogenic Shock	Coccygeal Ganglia

*The throat is not included because it is not a site of primary emotional **experience**, it is involved with **expression**, as are the face and hands.*

Table 2   **COMMON EXPRESSIONS AND REGIONS OF EXPERIENCE OF EMOTION**

Even though the connection between specific somatic affect and specific emotions has not been generally noted in the literature a number of psychotherapists have noted the awareness of the bodily experience of emotion in common expressions.

Common Expression	Emotions	Body Region
Gutless (Felt like) kicked in the gut Yellow belly No guts	Shame, Negative Confidence	Umbilicus
Full of Gall Venting your spleen Pissed Off	Anger, Fear	Epigastric/ Hypochondriac
Heartsick Broken-hearted Heartache	Sadness, Grief	Heart
Pucker Factor[6]	Mortal Terror	Perineum

---

[5] Migraine has not usually been considered to be a heart related disorder. The disclosure of the relationship came from the discovery that SHEN procedures performed around the heart during the migraine paroxysm often both ended the migraine and revealed deep-seated grief of long standing.

[6] Pucker Factor: Paratrooper's phrase, refers to a distinct bodily sensation noted when about to jump.

CHAPTER 3

RESULTS OF RELEASING PHYSIOEMOTIONAL TENSIONS IN
TWENTY-FIVE SHEN CASES

This chapter was originally published by the author as a paper titled: *"A Review of 25 Clinical Cases Suggestive of Anatomic Specificity in Psychosomatic and Somatoform Disorders and a Hypothesis for the Etiology and Treatment of These Disorders"*. The cases have been updated with current follow-up information, as was available.

CRITERIA
The cases presented in this paper were chosen for the imagery evoked, emotionality displayed or abreactive episodes[7] that were concomitant with the amelioration or cessation of pain and/or other symptoms. They were selected from a larger number of similar cases which resulted in reduction of symptoms and complaints, but did not produce the more vivid emotionality or memory shown in the cases selected for this paper. The results in these cases are confirmed by observations from hundreds of cases where the relaxation procedures, when performed on normal people without physical disorders, produced similar release of emotion specific to the region of application.

TREATMENT MODALITY
SHEN Physioemotional Release Therapy is a series of non-invasive touch relaxation techniques applied sequentially to the various regions of the body. In a high percentage of cases, application of SHEN at one of the specific regions in the body will induce far deeper relaxation then when SHEN is applied at other body regions. Deep relaxation is evidenced by changes in heart rate, breath rhythm and rate, myoclonic jerks and in various eye and mouth movements associated with sleep and dream states. In psychosomatic and somatoform disorders the deepest relaxation invariably occurs when the intervention is applied in the region encompassing the dysfunctioning organs. Usually, the treatment consists of a series of interventions spaced a day or two apart.

Frequently, REM or NREM is observed as emotionally charged dreams; overt emotion or abreaction occur during the deeper states.[8] Examination of the specific emotions reported by the patient shows significant pairings of specific organs and specific emotions, relationships previously unreported in the literature. The significance of these relationships in anatomic specificity is evident in the case histories.

---

[7] Abreactive episode: Vivid reliving of an event of personal importance. Often includes recall of sensations of sound, smell, taste and touch.

[8] The timing and location of release of the major somatic affect and memory/abreaction was independently validated by therapist and patient:

(a) Eye movement and breath rate were noted by the therapist. Sudden changes in breath rhythm and rate and occurrences of REM and NREM were taken as evidence of of the surfacing of the emotion or abreaction. The region of the body where the hands were placed when this occurred was noted.
(b) Spontaneous reports from the patients regarding placement of the hands when they lost wakefulness or felt a physiological sensation of some sort or recalled having the memory, validated the therapists observation of location.

PATIENT SELECTION

The patients were self selected, having appeared for treatment in the normal fashion, usually after having tried a range of treatments for the presenting disorders. A few patients selected themselves out before treatment was complete; these are noted. In some cases SHEN interventions were not the only treatment, however in those cases it appeared to be the pivotal one, because change in symptoms were reported during or immediately following the critical SHEN treatment.

CONSIDERATIONS OF SUGGESTIBILITY

Because the following cases were clinical, rather than research study cases, screening and tight controls for suggestibility and hysterical personality were neither appropriate or practical. It was felt that, since all patients had been treated by other methods without significant result, suggestibility was not a major controlling factor. Few of the patients evidenced belief in the method, some were, "Willing to try anything since nothing else worked" and some showed outright skepticism.

Suggestions as to expected effect were kept to the barest minimum. In many cases the patient was not advised that emotion or memory of forgotten events might occur. This led to some patient management problems when emotions occurred without warning. In most cases the emotions that surfaced seemed to surprise the patient.[9] Comments on individual suggestibility are noted for most of the cases.

THERAPISTS

Usually the patient had only one therapist, however in some cases more than one was involved. Therapists are identified as J, M, R, S, T, & V.

CLINICS

The cities are indicated as: A, Amarillo D, Dallas F, Fort Worth L, Las Vegas M, Milwaukee S, Sausalito.

ORGANIZATION OF CASES

The cases are grouped by disorders under the anatomical region where the intervention was performed. Number of cases per disorder is indicated.

LOWER GASTROINTESTINAL
Irritable Bowel Syndrome(2)
Multiple Abdom. Complaints(1)

UMBILICAL
Chronic Low Back Syndrome (6)

PUBIC/ILIAC
Premenstrual Syndrome (3)

HEART
Migraine (4)
Clustr Headache(1)
Chest Pain(1)
Hypertension(1)

EPIGASTRIC/HYPOCHONDRIAC
Eating Disorders (3)

PERINEUM
Coma/Psychognic Shock(1)
Post Traumatic Stress Dsrdr(1)
Night Terror (1)

---

[9] Sudden recall of forgotten events during or shortly following the procedure is not uncommon. Pertinent personal information surfaced in many cases. Much of this information was pivotal and had not previously been available.

THE CASE HISTORIES

INTERVENTIONS AT LOWER GASTROINTESTINAL REGION

DISORDER: MULTIPLE UNRELATED ABDOMINAL COMPLAINTS   **Cases Reviewed: 1**

CASE "A"
Patient: Female, 31 years.
Presenting Complaint: Chronic cystitus, chronic vaginitis, various recurring digestive complaints and frequent attacks of intestinal virus.
Clinic: A.
Therapist: R.

History: Refractory to numerous prescription medications and herbal remedies. Had not responded to a series of colonics, fasts, psychotherapy and primal therapy.

Considerable pain of shifting focus. At time of treatment pain in right hypochondrium and left iliac regions. Began sobbing and wailing forlornly during procedure (procedure does not cause pain of itself) with some release of gas. Sobbing intensified at both pain sites then diminished as pain resolved. By procedure's end pain disappeared and patient happened to recall being weaned suddenly and abruptly at two months. The next day patient reported feeling wonderful and spoke in a deep firm voice which was not evident before the treatment. Second treatment produced no further sobbing.

Fourteen months later patient reported, "I have not had any more trouble with that part of my body since you worked on me".

Suggestibility: Came for treatment at someone else's suggestion. Willing but expressed no particular expectation. Had not responded to any of her previous treatments, which she had believed would help her.

Last Contact: Five years after treatment.
Condition: Except for isolated flu, no recurrence of the ailments.

DISORDER: IRRITABLE BOWEL SYNDROME[10,11]   **Number of Cases Reviewed: 2**

CASE "B"
Patient: Female, age 43.
Presenting Complaint: Lower Back Pain, indigestion.
Clinic: F.
Therapist: T.
History: Bowel trouble entire life. Guilt about husband's death (three years prior). Guilt about not caring for mother (whom she was caring for). Felt entire responsibility even though other siblings had greater means. Angry about the guilt. Prescribed laxatives were taken regularly.

Treatment induced gut rumblings and flatulence provoking profuse mortification and apologies. Waves of anger and sadness followed treatment. Following second treatment, bowel loosened to near diarrhea.[12] After two days halted the laxatives and bowel assumed normal function for first time in years. Further treatments produced no further rumblings or flatulence. Back pain abated during the first treatment, ended after the second and did not return. Normal Bowel function continued.

Suggestibility: No suggestion was made that treatment might effect the gastroenteritis since this complaint was not known to the therapist.
Last Contact: 2 months
Condition: No back or bowel complaints. Reports being more assertive, less guilt, has separated farther from mother. No laxatives being taken.

CASE "C"
Patient: Male, age 52.
Presenting Complaint: Spastic Colon
Clinic: S.
Therapist: R.
History: Constant pain in right and left iliac for six months, from the time patient quit job because of stress. Colonic seizure during colonoscopy, at 30cm. At times pain became burning and spread to navel. Stools hard. No results from biofeedback. Dissatisfied with life.

Pain resolved during first treatment which induced eruptions of gas pockets. Spontaneously reported "Feeling much better about myself" the day following treatment. Bowel movements increased from once to twice a day for several days, then returned to normal with stools of a better consistency. Pain did not return. Second treatment produced only minor gas. Patient continued to feel better about himself, was clearly more cheerful and actively began to look for new career opportunities.

Suggestibility: "Heard good things about the treatment", eager to try. (No suggestion was made of possible change in self image.)
Last Contact: Six months.
Condition: Pain has not returned. Reports being able to detach from stressful situations in new job and is "Really feeling a lot better".

---

[10] *"...has long been a suspicion that patients with the irritable bowel or colon have emotional disorders as well"* p.318 Gastrointestinal Pathophysiology

[11] *"....rigidity, meticulousness, obsessive-compulsiveness, as well as emotional lability, lethargy and headaches have been associated with IBS".* p.263 Cecil Essentials of Medicine

[12] *"Diarrhea .... can be thought of as related to inhibition of phasic colon contractions ...."* p.66 Gastrointestinal Pathophysiology.

DISORDER: LOW BACK SYNDROME[13],[14]   **Number of Cases Reviewed: 6**

CASE "D"
Patient: Male, age 39
Presenting Complaint: Severe Lower Back Pain
Clinic: F.
Therapists: R, T, S.
History: Strained back during routine job operation. Laminectomy. Discs between S1/L4/L5 badly swollen. Papain injections ineffective.

First treatment was just prior to removal of discs S1-L4. pain abated.
Second treatment two months after the surgery. During treatment, REM occurred several times. Following treatment reported several memory flashes. One was of a fight with his father which he felt guilty about and the second was of proposing to his wife, while feeling that he would not be accepted. Pain abated considerably during treatment, but did not end. Reported feeling greater emotion than ever before. Subsequent treatments produced noticeable reductions in pain and continued to bring memory flashes, most related to self worth.

Suggestibility: Expressed considerable skepticism, but agreed to try.
Last Contact: Twenty months following second treatment.
Condition: No recurrence of pain, has had resolution with father.

CASE "E"
Patient: Male, age 42
Presenting Complaint: Chronic Low Back Pain
Clinic: F.
Therapist: R.
History: Strained lower back while lifting a small piece of machinery with another man. Laminectomy, S1-L2 seven years prior to treatment. Doing well until training for a new job, three months prior to treatment. Physical therapy and biofeedback not productive. Used walker with difficulty. Conversation filled with statements indicating extreme concern about "doing things right", being "extremely careful".

Painful to lie down for treatment. Awake throughout treatment which produced tears and the statement, "Grown men don't cry". "My wife would think its not manly to cry". Stated he felt unworthy and evidenced deep shame at somehow having failed. Pain lessened markedly during treatment but did not end. He walked (with walker) and breathed easier. Before second treatment, developed gastroenteritis, and withdrew from program.

Suggestibility: Extremely skeptical, but agreed to try.
Last Contact: No further contact
Condition: Unknown

---

[13] *"In many cases, an organic disorder reasonably accounts for the symptoms, but psychogenic factors become evident when symptoms and disability persist or worsen after the signs of injury or disease have cleared".* Merck Manual, 13th Ed.

[14] *"Anxiety causes muscle tension that leads to pain, which in turn leads to more anxiety, more muscle tension and more pain."* p.26 Clinical Symposia 32-6.

CASE "F"
Patient: Male age 32
Presenting Complaint: Constant Lower Back Pain Following Injury
Clinic: F.
Therapists: R, T.
History: Member police force. Fell on back onto a small projection during training. No evidence of physical damage. Currently on sick leave. Evidenced considerable concern about being able to continue to perform in his job, afraid he would be transferred to a lesser job if he couldn't get himself together.

Ten minutes into the treatment his back noticeably relaxed and he was in deep sleep. Awakened thirty minutes later, pain entirely gone. Minor pain developed around shoulders the next day which was temporary. Regular physical therapy workouts brought no recurrence of pain.

Suggestibility: Doubtful about success before treatment, startled when it produced results, expressed amazement.
Last Contact: 1 month
Condition: Back at work. No recurrence of pain in that region.

CASE "G"
Patient: Male, age 37.
Presenting Complaint: Back pain, limp
Clinic: F
Therapist: R
Treatment History: Back injured on job, two years prior, slow recovery. While training for new job was knocked onto hands and knees and a crane dropped a small load on his lower back. Pain resulted in laminectomy following accident. "Poor me" attitude. Conversation was filled with remarks about how badly life treated him. He was not paid properly, was required to do things he shouldn't have to do (in his opinion).

First treatment produced marked lessening of pain. Reported sleeping better, pain remained reduced for twenty four hours.

Fell asleep during second treatment. Shortly after waking appeared in the clinic's office, eyes wide, excitedly said "I just walked to the sink for a drink of water and when I got there I realized that I hadn't limped!"

Limp did not return. Energy level and excitement at life skyrocketed. Was able to do his prescribed physical therapy.

Suggestibility: Was clearly startled by the results of the treatment.
Last Contact: Two months after treatment
Condition: The reversal of personal attitude did not maintain. After a few weeks tremendous guilt feelings began to emerge and he developed severe digestive disorders. Did not return to clinic. However, limp and back pain had not recurred.

CASE "H"
Patient: Male, age 32.
Presenting Complaint: Chronic back pain
Clinic: S.
Therapist: R.
History: Long term low back pain. Entered hospital annually for 7-10 days of traction. Poor self image. Commented that "People say I don't take myself seriously". Often let others take advantage of him, agreed that he needed to stand up for himself. Short, banty rooster type.

During first treatment pain ended. Left amazed. Failed to keep second appointment. Upon contact advised that the pain had returned 24 hours later and "I don't want something that only works for 24 hours." Admitted that he had been told that two or three treatments would be necessary and agreed to return for additional treatments. During next treatment he woke, startled, and said "I just saw a black ball shrink to the size of a pea and fly out of my back". Pain ended completely. Was advised to take time to let his back regain its strength. He agreed.

Suggestability: Not very interested, came at the insistence of a relative. Expressed doubt.
Last Contact: Two months after last treatment.
Condition: He remained pain free for six weeks until he was asked to help move a refrigerator. Unable to stand up for his need to finish healing, he agreed, severely straining his back. Pain returned in force.

CASE "I"
Patient: Male, age 40.
Presenting Complaint: Severe Lower Back Pain
Clinic: L.
Therapist: R.
History: Episodes of back pain since childhood. Pain had become severe for last several months. Ate pain pills like candy. CAT scan negative. Patient demanded operation but fortunately his surgeon refused. Patient had recognized that back pain flared when he fought with his wife or when stress at work increased.

One treatment. His back relaxed markedly during treatment. After treatment he stated "I'm not going to say it doesn't hurt because you didn't do anything". After a few minutes he admitted having a memory. He refused to discuss it saying "You wouldn't believe it". Finally, he said, "I remembered being stabbed in the back, but nothing like that ever happened to me". Refused to discuss the pain further, or whether he still had pain. Shortly afterward, his co-workers reported that he had stopped taking his pain pills.

Six months later he happened to meet the therapist and when asked how the pain was snapped "What pain", and walked away.

Suggestibility: Highly skeptical, refused to believe treatment would help, even after it had.
Last Contact: Two years.
Condition: Co-workers report no further pain medication.

DISORDERS: PREMENSTRUAL SYNDROME[15,16,17]   **Number of Cases Reviewed: 3**
                & MENSTRUAL DISTRESS

CASE "J"
Patient: Female, 26 years.
Presenting Complaint: Premenstrual Syndrome with mild hypothyroidism
Clinic: S.
Therapist: R.

History: Irritability and vague unpleasantness prior to menses and pain during menses. Low energy, Thyroxin effect negligible. Child of mother who elected to bear children after developing MS. Patient recalled having to be quiet during play and to be conscious of mother's illness.
Patient wore dark, unfashionable clothing. Patient seemed almost transparent in a curious way. Functioned well, was quite efficient but never seemed to disturb the world as she went about her work and life.

Four treatments produced spectacular, spontaneous visions. First vision was her mother's face smiling at her, without warning the face became a viper and struck at her. During the next session an abreaction occurred. Patient relived standing outside her mother's parlor door, at age three, hearing mother say, "I never should have had the girls", to a friend. During next treatment a cartoonlike vision appeared and the patient burst out laughing, "I just saw my ovaries, they had little feet and one said to the other, *Now we can run,* and they ran off". The statement proved to be an accurate prediction.

Next ovulation and period arrived without discomfort. Within weeks she began wearing brighter, lighter weight and much more fashionable clothing. She began examining her life and relationships and proceeded to make major alterations in both. Her voice became stronger as well. Her menstrual discomfort did not return.

Suggestibility: Believed treatment could possibly help the PMS. However, no suggestion was made that the memory might occur. It was interesting that she had spontaneously mentioned prior to treatment that she "worked out all my stuff about my parents in therapy five years ago".

Last Contact: Four years after treatment
Condition: No recurrence of discomfort. Appears to be much stronger emotionally. Attitude with others is one of quiet confidence.

---

[15] *"..We have only a broad definition of this disorder, no set criteria for its diagnosis, and no treatment that has been demonstrated to be more effective than placebo. ... emotional symptoms are predominant in the syndrome... ."* p.785 Psychosomatics Oct. 1985, Vol. 26 No. 10.

[16] *"Psychological symptoms (of) Tension, Irritability, Depression, including lack of confidence and notions of unworthiness ... Poor emotional control, Illogical emotional reactions ... Low or absent sex drive"* from list, pp. 62,63 The Premenstrual Syndrome - Shreeve.

[17] *"Other researchers assert that PMS complaints are a way to express distress about environmental situations, difficulties in interpersonal relationships, personal attitudes about being a woman, and guilt over sexual temptation."* (Reid R.L. 1981) p.13 Behavioral medicine update V. 5 No. 4 1984.

CASE "K"
Patient: Female, age 38
Presenting complaint: Pain throughout back (Did not mention PMS)
Clinic: S.
Therapist: R.
History: Pain throughout back following accident two years prior. Difficulty sleeping. Biofeedback ineffective in lowering pain.

First session produced major lessening of pain. Second was during start of menses, however this was not mentioned until after the session which resulted in cessation of menstrual pain. Patient later reported that her period was the easiest she had ever had and expressed amazement at how wonderful she felt about herself.
Suggestibility: Biofeedback ineffective.
Last Contact: 6 months
Condition: "Periods still a lot easier." Cramping and pain less, not as depressed, "Amazed that I have so much energy during them."(menses)

CASE "L"
Patient: Female, age 38
Presenting Complaint: Severe Menstrual Bleeding
Clinic: M.
Therapists: M, R.
History: Excessive bleeding for four years. One year prior to divorce and three years following. Last four months severe bleeding, the last with large clots. Hemoglobin had dropped to 9 gms. D & C performed but bleeding did not halt, still clotting. Six days after D & C began progesterone. No bleeding during fourteen months on progesterone. Her physician advised her that her ovaries were not functioning.

First treatment one week before period produced deep sleep and image of decaying matter. Patient slept for two hours, got up and went to bed.

Second treatment three weeks later, just following her menstrual period, produced sensation of intense heat at ovaries, followed by feeling of coolness. Patient reported the area felt "clean and light".

Following treatment patient reported feeling a sense of self esteem for the first time since her marriage and that she had never felt self esteem except as part of the marriage partnership.

Patient began cutting back progesterone to half one month later. At the end of two more months had ended the progesterone entirely. The next two months saw her cycle returning to its original, stable 25 day cycle. First day of menses heavy flow, second day moderate, third day light, fourth day minor. Feels some tension first day only.

Suggestibility: Wanted the treatment to work. Claimed no special faith in the process as she was not familiar with it.
Last Contact: 17 months following last treatment.
Condition: Excellent. No recurrence of bleeding. Patient believes ovaries are functioning because she observes a clear discharge during the time when ovulation would occur.

DISORDERS: EATING DISORDERS   **Number of Cases Reviewed: 3**

CASE "M"
Patient: Female, 42 years
Presenting Complaint: Anorexia/Bulimia, Low Back Pain
Clinic: F
Therapists: R, S, T.
History: Typical bingeing and purging phases. Kleptomania since age 14.

Several treatments. First produced lessening of back pain and noticeable increase in range of motion in one direction. Second treatment further increased range of motion, pain ceased and she had an abreaction of the last time she had been caught shoplifting. (This memory had been lost to her conscious mind.) A later treatment produced another abreaction, of an early life situation that contributed to the onset of the disorders.

Suggestibility: Had been resistant to psychotherapy and biofeedback.
Last Contact: 4 months.
Condition: No further back pain, no physical complaints, nor episodes of eating and purging.

CASE "N"
Patient: Female, 27 years.
Presenting Complaint: Atypical Anorexia
Clinic: F
Therapists: R, S.

History: Stopped weighing herself when weight dropped past 89 pounds (Height 5'7"). Parental relationship distant and she was without appetite. Seeing a psychologist. Had actively pursued appropriate psychotherapies and biofeedback without effective result.

A significant SHEN treatment resulted in a series of frightening dreams and brief period of nausea. Appetite reawakened shortly and increased slowly over next few weeks. Her weight is now within normal and the once difficult parental relationship, according to both patient and delighted parents, is now resolved. There has been no recurrence of the anorexia. Indeed, is often the first one at the table, sometimes being chided for not waiting for all to be seated before starting to eat.

Suggestibility: Believed the technique might work, however she had believed biofeedback would be effective, but it had not been.[18]
Last Contact: Two years after treatment.
Condition: No recurrence, weight gain stable.

---
[18] Patient later revealed that she had not trusted the male therapist and therefore had believed she would not allow the therapy to work.

CASE "O"
Patient: Female, 24 years.
Presenting Complaint: Appetite loss following trauma
Clinic: S.
Therapists: J, R.

History: Severely burned in auto accident. Six weeks following accident had not regained appetite. No internal organ injuries. Unable to do more than nibble at her food.

One hour after first SHEN treatment ate a whole chicken breast, a few vegetables and part of a piece of chocolate cake. Anger about accident, which had never surfaced, began to emerge in her thoughts and dreams.

She was not normally expressive and had evidently suppressed anger on a number of occasions as considerable anger emerged following the second session. (Part of anger was toward her father which she demonstrated through transference to the older, male therapist who had treated her, by insisting that he had done everything wrong.) Appetite rapidly improved to normal. The release of anger brought with it some valuable insights which were absorbed.

Suggestibility: Extremely doubtful about treatment. Had to be cajoled by a friend to try it. Did so on the grounds that it might help her pain. For a time denied effectiveness in spite of appetite increase.

Last Contact: 22 months after treatment.
Condition: No recurrence of pain, appetite continues normally.

INTERVENTIONS AT HEART REGION

DISORDER: HYPERTENSION   **Number of Cases Reviewed: 1**

CASE "P"
Patient: Male, Age 43.
Presenting Complaint: High Blood Pressure, Shoulder pain.
Clinic: S.
Therapist: R.

History: On medication for BP of 180/118.

Following second treatment abreaction occurred during the night involving a close relative who had recently died. Woke to find pillow wet with tears. Shoulder pain gone. Admitted that he had not been able to grieve at the time of death because of pressures of the moment.   Blood pressure dropped to near normal.

Suggestibility: Successful Businessman, did not appear suggestible.
Last Contact: 7 years following treatment.
Condition: No recurrence of shoulder pain or high blood pressure. Blood pressure ranges around 120/80, no medication.

DISORDER: CHEST PAINS   **Number of Case Histories: 1**

CASE "Q"
Patient: Male, age 27
Presenting symptom: Chest Pain
Clinic: S.
Therapist: R.

History: Chest pains for four years. No evidence of heart trouble. Reported difficulty relating with women and deep desire for a relationship. Appeared tense, drawn.

Two treatments ended the chest pains. Next contact was a year later, patient was relaxed and relationship desires were not troubling him. Was clearly a much warmer, friendlier person.

Suggestibility: Unknown.
Last Contact: Five years after treatment.
Condition: No further chest pains.

DISORDER: MIGRAINE[19,20]   **Number of Cases Reviewed: 4**

CASE "R"
Patient: Female, 36 years
Presenting Complaint: Migraine
Clinic: F
Therapists: R, T.
History: Married eight years. History of physical and mental abuse during marriage.

Treatments at the heart region produced deep relaxation. Release of tears and sadness following treatment. Began to have a more positive attitude about herself. No further migraines while in hospital.

Suggestibility: Unknown
Last contact: 9 months
Condition: Separated from husband. No further migraine, still more assertive.

CASE "S"
Patient: Male, Age 53.
Presenting Complaint: Migraine
Clinic: S.
Therapist: R.
History: Occasional migraine episodes. Patient arrived during severe episode. Insisted on lying down during questioning as pain was too intense for him to stand up. Not on medication. Reported being out of work and without a place to live.

Patient began snoring ten minutes into treatment. On awakening reported no migraine, but minor occipital pain. Patient left and promptly entered heavy freeway traffic, but migraine did not return and occipital pain ended shortly. Following the half hour drive, was very sleepy and napped for about an hour. Reported feeling much better the next day.

Suggestibility: Came at recommendation of friend, difficult to asses suggestibility because of severity of pain at beginning of visit. Nonplussed that pain had ended.
Last Contact: 6 months.
Condition: No migraines, some other headache.

---

[19] The SHEN intervention for migraine is performed at the lower heart region and at the aortic arch. Deeply repressed grief has frequently surfaced during this procedure. Grief is usually closely linked with anger. Since sadness is experienced at the central heart region and anger at the lower heart region (Solar Plexus) it is easy to see that the emotional linkage is paralleled by organ linkage.

[20] *"Fromm-Reichman (1937) concluded from experience with eight patients that 'they could not stand to be aware of their hostility against beloved persons; therefore they unconsciously tried to keep this mostly repressed and finally expressed it by the physical symptoms of the migraine.'"* p. 403 Wolf's Headache, 4th edition.

CASE "T"
Patient: Female, 34 years.
Presenting Complaint: Migraine
Clinic: F.
Therapist: T.
History: Under treatment for years. Treatment included Biofeedback and some Psychotherapy. Hospitalized for the Migraine. Attacks since age nine, occurring weekly or biweekly, lasting 3 to 4 days. Onset almost always on Wednesday. Could not remember emotional trauma at age nine.

First treatment was on a Tuesday. During treatment patient dropped into deep sleep with REM. Shortly after awakening "just happened" to recall that her parents had divorced when she was nine and that she had almost drowned that same year. Expected attack on Wednesday did not occur.

Asked therapist if treatment would help her nightmares. When questioned she stated, "I've had them ever since I can remember, I used to crawl in bed with my parents when I'd get them".

Patient revealed that she was married to a wife beater who had recently broken her jaw. Three other treatments during the next two weeks, no further migraine.

Suggestibility: Unknown, but had been doing biofeedback to no avail.
Last Contact: Six months following last treatment
Condition: No recurrence of migraine. Reported that she had divorced her husband in the interim.

CASE "U"
Patient: Female, age 26.
Presenting Complaint: Migraine.
Clinic: D.
Therapists: R, V.
History: Frequent migraines for previous five months. No pattern. Sudden, intense, patient would faint and fall, sometimes with injury.

One treatment. Produced REM while intervention was at aortic arch. After session therapist asked if anything significant had occurred the month prior to the beginning of the attacks. She replied, "My mother had heart surgery". When asked where, on her mothers body it was performed, she drew a line precisely across the aortic arch and said, "She had five bypasses, here"[21].

Patient revealed that she was last of six girls and that her mother wanted her to get married and produce grandchildren. Patient wanted to go into business for herself, instead.

Suggestibility: Very skeptical, agreed because co-workers insisted.
Last Contact: Two months following treatment.
Condition: One mild attack. Quit job to go into business for herself.

---

[21] This case probably could be classified as a transpersonal conversion disorder.

DISORDER: CLUSTER HEADACHE   **Number of Cases Reviewed : 1**

CASE "V"
Patient: Female, age 30
Presenting Complaint: Cluster Headache
Clinic: S.
Therapist: R.
History: Series of Clusters for preceding six weeks. Ergotamine sometimes effective. Upper body damp with sweat. Patient remarked that "It feels like razors down my spine." (Indicated they ended where the skin dampness ended, at the papillary muscle.)

Treatment performed at the papillary muscle as attack was building. Headache ended within three minutes and did not return. Deep personal grief surfaced.

Subsequently, on four or five occasions the attacks began but subsided as the patient intentionally tried to relax that area.

Suggestibility: Patient was aware of the treatment modality, but also knew that it had never been used for cluster headaches.
Last Contact: Two years after treatment.
Condition: No full blown attacks, only mild beginnings.

INTERVENTIONS AT PERINEUM REGION[22]

DISORDER: COMA COMPLICATED BY PSYCHOGENIC SHOCK   **Number Cases Reviewed:1**

CASE "W"
Patient: Male, Age 14.
Presenting Complaint: Coma
Clinic: S.
Therapist: R.
History: Struck by bus, suffered blood clot on brain. Operation successful, but patient remained in steady, restless coma for eight days. Minimal response to external stimuli.

Single treatment at perineum resulted in two brief (five to six second) manifestations of fear including terrified moans and thrashing of arms. Patient drifted off to relaxed sleep. Within six hours woke and was sitting up in a chair talking to people. Recovery proceeded swiftly.

Suggestibility: Not a factor. Patient was not aware of treatment and has no recall of the treatment.
Last Contact: Three years.
Condition: No relapse.

---

[22] The somatic affect of Mortal Fear presents in the body at this region, producing a contraction that is often painful. One can imagine that the effect of contraction around the caudal ganglia would necessarily affect the entire sympathetic nervous system thus impairing virtually all body functions. Mortal fear is quite different in both quality and location from the experience of ordinary, common fear, such as the fear of being late to work.

DISORDER: POST TRAUMATIC STRESS DISORDER   **Number of Cases Reviewed: 1**

CASE "X"
Patient: Female, age 25.
Presenting Complaint: Post Traumatic Stress Disorder
Clinic: F.
Therapists: R, T, S.
History: Injured in accident five years prior. Broken L. Clavicle, three broken ribs, ruptured Spleen, broken L. Pelvis, broken L. Leg, all healed. Dazed look - eyes slightly glassy, fixed smile, shuffling walk, rigid body, flat affect. Multiple body pains, constant headache since accident. No recall of accident in spite of several attempts through hypnosis. Autogenic training, Biofeedback and physical therapy had not lessened pain. Prognosis did not suggest improvement.

This was a difficult case and involved some twenty-five treatments extending over three months. Her symptoms eroded slowly and by three months head pain had been absent for two weeks and she had experienced three flashes of recall (including fear) about the accident, her body pains were minimal, she laughed and/or was angry as appropriate and her face was no longer fixed in a smile. Her skin had regained its color and her eyes were no longer glassy. Range and ease of motion were near normal. She arrived for treatment one day and announced, "Now that I don't have pain any longer I guess I'll be going off welfare. I think I want to go back to college so I'm planning to take a course at beauty college to support myself through school." Which she did.

Suggestibility: Did not appear high. Had tried everything and was willing to do whatever was suggested. Seemed resigned to her condition.
Last Contact: Two years after treatment
Condition: Some headache began about two months after entering beauty college. Seemed due to standing all day. Relieved by light traction.

DISORDER: NIGHT TERRORS   **Number of Cases Reviewed: 1**

CASE "Y"
Patient: Male, 10 months
Presenting Complaint: Night Terrors
Clinic: S.
Therapist: R.
History: Unable to sleep more than 3 hours without waking screaming. Extremely dependent on mother. Continuous since birth without let up.

Child was treated while asleep. Intervention performed only at root. Child woke, screaming just prior to third treatment, treatment performed for three minutes when child stopped screaming. Therapist left, child was sniffling with his thumb in his mouth. This was the last of his night terrors. (Night terror is not psychosomatic but the episodes could be related to birth trauma, and therefore PSTD. It is also possible the child had episodes of bowel pain. The case is included because of the association of terrifying fear at the perineum.)

Suggestibility: No possibility
Last Contact: 2 years after treatment.
Condition: Within a week he began brief temper tantrums and making demands. Parents were delighted. The terror never returned.

From these and many other cases which support the concept, we make the observations:

(1) The underlying cause of the physiological disorders was long-term involuntary repression of painful somatic affect.

(2) It appears that continuous repression of specific somatic affect results in specific organ dysfunction. In the cases reviewed, each emotion was associated with only a small range of disorders. Thus it appears that instead of affecting the body generally, stress is regional in nature having both regional cause and regional result.

Figure 2 SOMATIC EFFECTS OF SOME REPRESSED EMOTIONS

Repression of the emotion of:

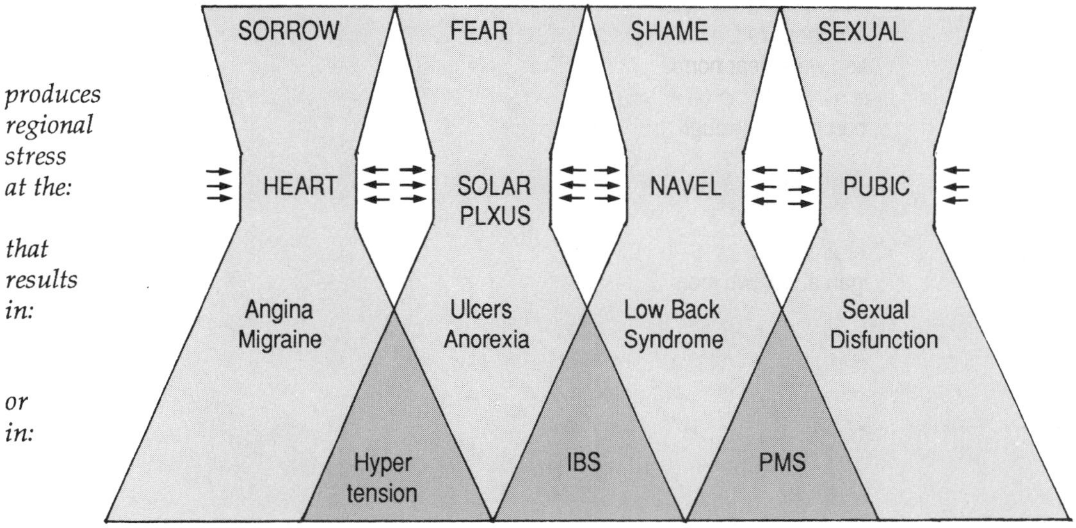

where the contractile stresses combine in adjacent, overlapping regions.

It is presumed that when stress caused by a single dominant emotion results in general, body-wide effects, it is because the regional stress has affected one or more organs or glands that have wide-ranging systemic effects. (Thus, the systemic effects during premenstrual syndrome that are caused by changes in body levels of estrogen or progesterone are due to tensions surrounding the ovaries.)

(3) It is only painful somatic affects that are associated with physical dysfunction. Those somatic affects coupled with love, joy and confidence did not surface during these cases.

(4) Once free of the contractile tension, the patients were free to live a fuller, more emotionally responsive life (which most of them did) and their bodies were no longer troubled by the effects of those tensions.

(5) Once the emotion was experienced, the trouble ended or reduced dramatically. This suggests that it is not the experience of the emotion that is the culprit but the repression of the emotion.

REVIEW OF

CHAPTERS 2 and 3

1. The effect of contractility focuses around:
   a. The center of body mass.
   b. The extremities.
   c. The pain site.
   d. The epicenter of the body.

2. The Splinting Reflex
   a. Is an involuntary reaction.
   b. Covers a wound with tiny "splints" of tissue.
   c. Takes place after a broken bone is splinted.
   d. Is an effort by the conscious mind.

3. Regional Stress refers to:
   a. The different background stress levels in different countries.
   b. The differences between stress zones in this country.
   c. Stress results in specific body zones.
   d. The carryover from a stressful day.

4. Somatic Affect is:
   a. The effects of thinking about emotion.
   b. What we feel in the body when we feel emotion.
   c. The result of testing body reflexes under stress.
   d. A device to test the Physioemotional Field.

CHAPTER 4

BIOLOGICAL CONSEQUENCES OF CONTRACTILITY

From the range of cases affected by contractility it is evident that a large number of biological changes and effects occur during and following SHEN. Many of the cases involved the effects of tension on a gross level; on straight muscle tissue as in the cases of chronic low back pain but others, such as some of the eating disorders, involved a change in biochemical levels. Changes in appetite indicate a change in quantity of gastric juices and changes in ovulation and menstrual bleeding indicate changes in the biochemical output of the ovaries. While it has not been possible to measure the change in quantity or makeup of the biochemicals in those cases, it has in another situation. Several times hospitalized chemotherapy patients with severely lowered white blood counts have had marked increases in white count following SHEN treatments. These disorders all involve different organs and glands. There is nothing at all similar about the chemistry produced in these different glands and organs, nor are the chemical pathways the same.

It is clear that several **different** biochemical changes takes place in these disorders. The question is, what is the mechanism that causes the changes and how is it affected by SHEN? It is difficult to imagine how the relaxation of straight muscle tissue could account for these changes as it does with chronic low back pain. And it is even more difficult to support the idea that the composition or quantity of these biochemicals is directly affected by the physioemotional energy field. It is more likely that the effect would be through a physiological mechanism that is common to all the organs and glands.

There is a mechanism that fits these requirements, and its biological makeup closely approximates that of the straight muscle tissue which SHEN is known to affect. Even though the parenchyma (the individual functioning cells) are different in each of the organs and glands, their nourishment and waste disposal networks are identical. These networks are the capillaries, minute connecting tubules between the arterioles and the venules that are present in all body tissue.

CAPILLARY PERFUSION
The blood moving through the capillaries passes by the parenchyma dropping off nourishment and picking up waste metabolites. This flow is vital.[23] Flow through the capillaries is governed, in part, by pre-capillary sphincters. These doughnut shaped sphincters encircle the entrance to the capillary and are composed of a single smooth muscle cell. The sphincters open and close, as needed, to provide adequate normal blood perfusion. Normally they are closed, being opened perhaps five to ten percent of the time. Continuous, abnormal tensing of these sphincters would cause organ dysfunction, both by starving the cells and by accumulation of waste metabolites.

SHEN work has shown conclusively that body tissue becomes tense at the site of emotional suppression in the body. It seems likely that continuous tension in the region of emotion would effect the local precapillary (smooth muscle) sphincters, just as it does

---

[23] *"...this nourishment, or lack of it, is the cause of many, if not most disease states."* From the Introduction, Capillary Perfusion in Health and Disease, Hardaway, R.M.

with straight muscle tissue, causing them to remain closed more than they should. The parenchyma of the glands and organs in the region would then be poorly nourished and waste metabolites would accumulate. Either result would account for mild to severe organ dysfunction.

PROVING THE HYPOTHESIS
It has not been possible to prove that the precapillary sphincters are directly affected by the SHEN flows but there are several effects of SHEN that support the concept.

Reduction of swollen tissue. When SHEN treatments are performed at areas of swollen tissue, the swollen areas release fluid and noticeably reduce in size. *Sometimes this can be quite dramatic. I recall once doing a SHEN flow through a man's leg. The leg was in a cast from ankle to knee, having been broken two weeks before. When I finished he excitedly exclaimed, "My gosh, I can move my leg". The swollen leg which had tightly filled the cast had reduced enough to be able to move slightly.* This outcome is quite easy to substantiate with calipers.

Now, there are only two drainage pathways in body tissue that could account for this effect, the lymph system and the venous return system which is fed by the capillaries. Of these two, the venous return is far faster. It is most unlikely that the lymph system could account for the reduction of swelling simply because it doesn't function that rapidly. The idea that venous return is the responsible factor is supported by a consistent observation.

One of the effects noticed by SHEN practitioners is that they will often feel the temperature of their receiving hand[24] rise suddenly as the flow of energy passes through the person's body into their hand. This sudden increase usually occurs three to four seconds following a physiological reaction (REM, myoclonic jerks, etc) in the patient. This heat rise has been measured with sensitive gauges at plus or minus one degree fahrenheit. The only known way for skin temperature to increase is through an increase in capillary perfusion. This could only occur if the precapillary sphincters were opened more frequently, or for longer periods.

ORGANIC FACTORS IN TENSION
It seems probable that constant physioemotional tension affects the body adversely by reducing blood circulation and (possibly) lymph flow. With the blood (and/or lymph flow) reduced, those organs subjected to physioemotional tensions would simply fail to function properly and become more vulnerable to invasion by bacterial or viral agents.

If this is the case, then the improvement of organ and gland function that is noted following SHEN would be explained by relaxation of the precapillary muscle sphincters that control the capillaries, and the resultant improved blood flow.

---

[24] "Sending" and "Receiving" hands will be explained in the next section.

CHAPTER 5

APPROACHES TO DYSFUNCTION:
PSYCHOSOMATIC VERSUS INVOLUNTARY CONTRACTION

THE PSYCHOSOMATIC CONCEPT

In the conventional approach to "Psychosomatic" Disorder the patient is presumed to be mentally unhealthy, at least in part. The patient is seen to be subconsciously antagonistic to the doctor or psychologist. The patient's symptoms are split apart during treatment with biological treatment aimed at the local site of the presenting physiological symptoms and psychological treatment aimed at (emotions in) the brain. Good results are difficult to achieve, as soon as one disorder is cured it is followed by a new one in a continuing psychosomatic cycle.

THE CONCEPT OF CONTRACTILITY

Involuntary tensions developed in the body to contain painful somatic affect are the cause of organic and glandular dysfunction. Therefore, it follows that the patient is mentally healthy but with a body that is adversely affected by localized, suppressed emotion. The patient is considered to be in concordance with his doctor and/or psychologist's intentions.

The patient's symptoms are not split apart during treatment with biological treatment aimed at the local body site and the emotional treatment focused on the head. Site-Specific treatment is directed at deep relaxation of local tissue at the site of the suppressed emotion, the site of the dysfunctioning organ. When the local tension ends, organic dysfunction ends. **Biological treatment and emotional treatment are the same.**

THE PATIENT AND CONTRACTILITY

The patient will likely find favor with this approach. The view that psychosomatic disorder is subconsciously intentional is so poorly received by most patients that it is usually not suggested by the physician. Most patients are violently opposed to the idea that it is "all in their heads" when they perceive it to be "all in their bodies".

(This is not to say that deliberate, subversive attempts are not made by the occasional patient/client receiving SHEN. Often they are, but after all, no therapeutic intervention can be expected to prevail in the face of a powerful secondary gain. However, when no current benefit is being derived from a disorder caused by involuntary contractions, rapid and permanent results can be expected through release of these tensions.)

Diagrams of the two approaches are shown on the following two pages

Figure 3

PSYCHOSOMATIC BRAIN/BODY PATHWAYS

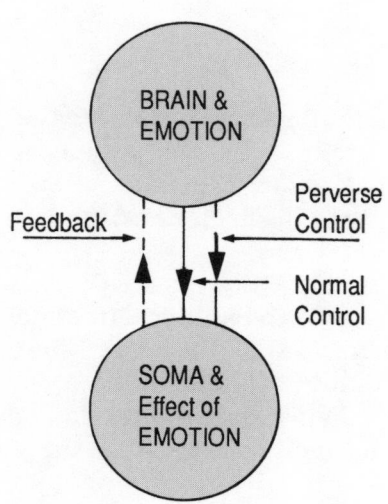

Biofeedback and/or Positive Thinking should be highly effective in altering the emotional state.

Emotion is thought to be developed and stored in the brain with its effects presenting in the body.

According to this model normal feedback from the body is "I hurt, now fix me". Part of the subconscious brain responds with appropriate corrective signals while
Another part of the subconscious sends perverse, counterproductive signals.

The result is garbled and nonproductive.

In this model the patient's subconscious is presumed to be in conflict with his conscious intentions and with his/her doctor or therapist.

Health is difficult to attain and maintain from this perspective

Figure 4

INVOLUNTARY BRAIN/BODY PATHWAYS

Positive Thought and Biofeedback affect normal biological control signals but have little effect on emotion. Helpful but hindered by suppressed emotion.

Emotion is produced experienced and then stored in the body.

Therefore, emotion locally suppressed in the body will directly and adversely affect local muscle and organ function.

In this model normal feedback includes both emotional feedback and biological feedback. The brain sends appropriate signals to try to correct the **biological** cause, but without effect, if the cause is emotion suppressed in the body.

However releasing the suppressed emotion will remove and correct the cause.

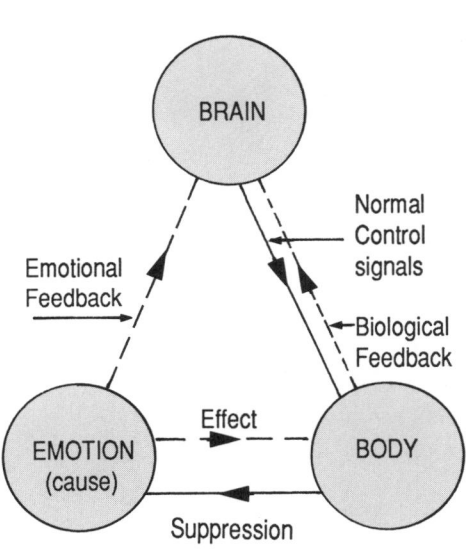

In this model the patient is not in dichotomy with himself or herself and is not a subconscious adversary to his/her doctor or therapist.

This is a model in which health can be attained and maintained.

REVIEW OF

CHAPTERS 4 and 5

1. Describe Contractility

2. How do you think patients would respond to the concept of contractility?

3. Which system, blood or lymph, does contractility affect most?

4. What is capillary perfusion?

*An emotion is impossible to define until you have
experienced it, and then you don't need to.*

CHAPTER 6   **EMOTION AND PHYSICS** _____ *39*
   The Two Basic Effects of Emotion, 40.   Body Movement in Relation to Emotion, 40.   Perception of Somatic
   Location of Emotion, 41.   Differing Stress Results of Different Emotions, 42.   Composition of Emotion -
   Biochemical? or Something Else?, 42.

   Review of Chapter 6, 44.

CHAPTER 7   **FIELD-LIKE EFFECTS OF EMOTION** _____ *45*
   Feeling Emotions of Others, 45.   Pheromones, 46.   The Mental Model of Emotion, 47.   Differences
   between Thoughts and Emotions, 47.   Rational Thought, 49.   Confusion? or Confused Thought?, 50.
   Biochemical Model of Emotion, 51.   The Fight or Flight Response, 52.   Examining the Experience of Fear,
   53.   The Energy Field Model of Fight or Flight, 54.   Which Came First? Emotion or Biochemical Change, 54.
   The Field Theory of Emotion, 55.

   Review of Chapter 7, 56.

CHAPTER 8   **PHYSICS OF THE PHYSIOEMOTIONAL FIELD** _____ *57*
   The Question of Evidence, 57.   Establishing the Nature of the Field, 58.   Other Experiments, 59.
   Organization and Pattern of the Flows, 61.   The Three Part Pattern, 64.   Field Action at the Emotion
   Centers, 66.   Some Difficult Questions, 70.

   Review of Chapter 8, 72.

UNRAVELING THE PUZZLE OF EMOTION

Emotion has always been a puzzle. It is difficult to sort out and understand its effects and it is just as difficult to control them. Most often, emotion is treated as an obstreperous child: don't spend too much time trying to understand it, just wait until it grows up and goes away. Because of this attitude, emotion has been denied the understanding of its place in the scheme of things.

Emotion is rarely ever studied by and for itself. There are hundreds of scientific societies, academies and research organizations for the investigation of every conceivable facet of medicine, psychology and biology but, as of this writing, none for the study of emotion, per se.

When emotion has been investigated at all it has been studied from only two orientations, the biochemical model and/or the mental model. Each of these models presumes emotion to be a subordinate and/or end process in its particular schema. However, both of these models have serious deficiencies, not only failing to answer many of the questions they intend to answer but raising new questions because of their conclusions.

We have been taught to view emotion as a result rather than a cause, but when we examine it carefully, we begin to suspect that this is not true, that emotion may be autonomous, an essence unto itself, an affecting factor in our lives that stands equal to the biological and the mental.

Indeed, emotion appears to be the primary controlling factor in our lives rather than a secondary one. It is the "stuff", or essence, that causes psychogenic and/or psychosomatic disorders and it is festering, uncompleted emotions that cause our thoughts to go in an "uncontrolled" direction in spite of our best intentions. *How could emotion be so dominant if it were merely an offshoot of the biological or of the mental?*

CHAPTER 6

THOUGHTS ON THE ESSENCE OF EMOTION

Somehow "emotion" seems to have slipped through a crack in the floor of the research laboratory. Virtually everything about emotion has been rigorously examined and subjected to the most minute scrutiny with one exception, *the nature of emotion itself.*

Psychological profiles address the results of emotions by using terms such as "poor self image" or "rigid personality" without regard to the specific emotions that produced those profiles. What happened to the "feeling sick with shame" or the "feeling worthless" that the person experienced in their gut? "Poor self image" and "rigid personality" are mental constructs, judgments, not the descriptions of emotions.

The biochemist discovers that epinephrine levels rise during a state of fear and promptly decides that the body has diverted blood from the epigastric region to the extremities because we don't need to digest food right then, we need to either fly or fight. But don't the muscles that activate the diaphragm need blood just as much as the extremities? Or could some other factor be involved in the shifting of blood volume? Could that factor have anything to do with mutual location, since the diaphragm/epigastric region is the region where we feel fear?

And for that matter, just what *is* fear - or any other emotion? Are emotions merely the result of a group of rationalized perceptions with biochemical overtones? Or does the way in which we feel emotions indicate that they might be something more than rationalization and/or chemistry?

No one would deny the implications of the autonomic, endocrine and limbic systems in the total effects and experience of emotion, but are any of these systems the cause of emotion or are they all merely responding to emotion? The evidence linking psychological underpinnings with an increasing range of somatic complaints mounts at the same time that increased research into possible neurological and endocrine causes fails to produce anything much beyond frustration. Certainly little resembling cures for these ailments has been uncovered.

It seems to me that the failure to make any real progress in linking psyche and soma in *psychosomatic* stems from the failure to recognize that emotions are not just accessories to, or byproducts of, brain function, but stand apart from both the biological brain and the biophysical body.

Emotions give every evidence that they are autonomous, essences unto themselves that interface between the body and the brain.

EMOTIONAL EXPERIENCE AND EMOTIONAL EXPRESSION

THE TWO BASIC EFFECTS OF EMOTION

The **expression** of emotion is distinctly different from the **experience** of emotion. The experience of emotion is what one **feels** and the expression of emotion is what one **does** as a result of that experience. Experience involves **inward sensation**, while expression involves **outward action**.

Expression of emotion involves (1) motion (2) occurs in the periphery of the body and (3) produces a physical **sensation** rather than an emotional feeling. (The sensation of moving one's hand is entirely different from the feeling of sadness, or of any other emotion.) Thus, expression of emotion is seen in shoulder shrugs, mouth movements, hand clenches, foot and leg jerks and eye blinks or squints.

Experience of emotion involves (1) somatic feelings which (2) cluster in five specific regions (3) central to the torso but (4) does **not** involve body motion. There are distinctively different "feelings", or **somatic affects** for the several different emotions. Feelings of love and sadness are experienced in the region of the heart, anger and most fear at the solar plexus, confidence, guilt, shame at the supranavel region, sexual arousal at the pubic region with physical fear, mortal terror appearing at the groin/perineum.

Conversion of Experience into Expression. The normal state of emotion is to produce **experience**. If allowed to expand, the experience or feelingness of the emotion becomes greater and greater. In spite of what many people think, *No body motion is required for this process*. However, if the **experience** of emotion is repressed or suppressed the effect, or force, of the emotion converts into **expression**. If we bottle up rage, for example, it converts into movement and something in our periphery reacts: a hand strikes out, a foot kicks or the mouth and vocal cords shape sounds and words.

BODY MOVEMENT IN RELATION TO EMOTION

1. The farther one gets from the emotion "centers" the more motion is observed during the event of an emotion. That is, expression of emotion involves little or no motion on the torso midline, more at the face and head, and even more with the hands and feet.

2. In spite of the fact that each emotion has a very specific feeling that is unique to it and it alone, the various motions resulting from (produced by) emotions are not specific to the various emotions. For example, the mouth may twitch in fear, in anger, or in the beginnings of joy, the toe may tap in disgust or anger or when startled in fear. There does not seem to be a specific emotional/neural activity for individual motions since all emotions can and will trigger very similar responses.

3. When the experience of emotional feeling at any of these regions is repressed and diverted into physical expression, or motion, it is as if motion leaves the midline and moves to the extremities. In fact, motion at the midline sometimes virtually ceases, as when near breath stoppage accompanies this diversion during the experience of fear. This is quite understandable; it requires tension to repress the emerging emotion and emphatic tension would necessarily halt body motion at that site.

Therefore, when one sees physical motion cues in a person, the cues are not so much evidence of **emotion** as evidence of **repression of emotion**. This includes crying, sobbing, and screaming. The more the emotional regions in the body are relaxed, the less vocal action takes place, even in the presence of very large emotion.

PERCEPTION OF SOMATIC LOCATION OF EMOTION

The site(s) of emotion(s) in the brain/body continuum is a matter of some conjecture. According to most theory, what we experience as emotion is merely a reflection of something that actually occurs in the brain, something that is reflected in the body through various neural and/or biochemical activities. This is a convenient supposition but one that wobbles badly in the face of serious questioning.

Subjective knowledge, of course, tells us that emotion is something in the torso. (This is universally true for all people but may not be noted by those whose torso is so blocked with defensive armor that they have no subjective emotional experiences, only the mental concomitants.)

Concurrence of Perceptions. Of course, the fact that I "feel" emotions in the various torso locations does not prove that they are indeed there and perhaps they are not. But I notice that with other perceptions this relationship between site of sensation and site of origin is accurate. If I feel a sharp pain in my finger I look at my finger to see why it hurts. If I cut my ankle I feel it in my ankle. The fact that I observe and record the event in my brain does not prevent me from recognizing that it occurred somewhere else.

Why should I not suppose that this relationship is accurate for the emotions as well as for other bodily sensations? Either the brain/body sensory perception of location is consistent or there are two systems, one that is accurate and one that is consistently confusing us with false perceptions as to the origin and loci of the emotions.

Logic. Looking at it from the other perspective, we could ask; "If I am experiencing something that is occurring in my brain, why do I not perceive it to be in my brain? Is there a reason for me to experience it elsewhere?" But there seems to be no reason. Indeed, there are times when it would be better if the perception were in the brain as experiencing emotion in the torso sometimes works counter to our best interests. One instance of this is during the experience of fear at the solar plexus. When large amounts of fear are experienced it becomes extremely difficult to breath, (See page 9). To breathe at all takes great effort and internal counselling, at precisely the time when we need to breathe the most. (Granted that some, when faced with the same situations, do not report difficulty breathing. But, when they do not, they do not report feeling fear, either.)

Clearly, if this is the result of a false perception, the effect is counterproductive, perhaps fatally so. In the situation given, it would be much better for optimum functioning to "feel" the emotion in the brain. *If the perception that fear is in the abdomen is a misplaced perception, there is something quite wrong with the arrangement.*

There seems to be no sensible need for the experience of emotion to be perceived in the body unless it is there. Logical sense tells us that emotion is experienced in the torso because that is just where it is.

THE DIFFERING STRESS RESULTS OF DIFFERENT EMOTIONS

Most research on "stress" has been on whole body functions. From this perspective any and all external situations are understood as producing stressors which **affect the entire body**. Any variances in the specific results obtained from person to person have been explained (or not explained) as anomalies or as "genetic or psychological predispositions". This perspective does not address the effects that the specific emotions evoked in any given situation might have on specific organs in the body.

But stress is never the same from situation to situation. Sadness, fear, shame all produce stress and the results are different for each of these emotions. Each stressful situation produces its own emotion or unique combination of emotions with one or two of these emotions becoming the dominant stressors. *It is the dominant emotion(s) in any stressful situation that determine the resultant somatic reaction/disorder.*

Emotional differences in stress. The reason there is a difference in the results of stress is because the individual emotions appear at different regions in the body. *This means that the stress of an emotion will affect its own somatic region more than any other.*

The mechanism is simple; repressing the unwanted somatic affect of an emotion requires physiological tension. For example, one stops the unpleasant feeling of fear by stopping breathing and one stops the feeling of shame by clenching the gut. (Conversely, increasing breath rate amplifies fear, a fact well known to breath therapists.) *Repression of individual emotions requires tension that largely affects the glands, organs and muscle tissue at one region alone.* The result is different syndromes for the different emotions.

Thus, repression of shame (in the region encompassing L4/L5/S1 and the ovaries) results in premenstrual syndrome and chronic low back syndrome, repression of grief (in the heart and chest) results in asthma and heart disorders and repression of anger (the region of the stomach and duodenum) results in ulcers. (We should note that these repressed emotions may not be justly earned emotions.)

COMPOSITION OF EMOTION - BIOCHEMICAL? OR SOMETHING ELSE?

It has often been assumed that the bodily sensations associated with emotions are the result of some reaction or change in body chemistry. However, not only is there no evidence to support this idea, there is considerable evidence to suggest that it is incorrect.

1. The subjective feeling states of the various emotions are mutually different. The feeling state, or somatic affect, of love is quite different from anger, which in turn is different from fear, from sadness, from shame etc. These differences are widely substantiated.

In addition, the feeling tone, as well as the somatic affect of some emotions is subtle but with others is quite dramatic. The quieter emotions, such as the feeling states of security, worthiness and achievement are subtle in sensory tone, induce a relaxed abdominal state *and do not upset normal biological functioning.* The more dramatic emotions, such as anger, fear and shame, jar the body, shake it out of its complacent stance and cause change in its biological function.

2. If emotions were indeed biochemical, then each emotion would have to have a unique biochemistry, as one biochemical compound could hardly produce these widely different feeling states.

3. The endocrine, autonomic and limbic pathways that are deeply implicated in the involvement of emotion with the body do not provide for biochemical differences of this sort. In order for there to be different chemistries, one or more of these systems would have to selectively activate the specific glands or organs that would be necessary to provide the specifically different biochemistry for each different emotion. There are, however, no glands or organs that have been shown to be the sources for the several individual emotions. (The heart, is popularly identified with love and sadness, not because it is known to produce any specific emotion-chemistry, but because those feelings are experienced at the heart region.) No chemistry has been discovered that can cause love, fear, shame or any of the other emotions.

4. The drugs that are available to alter "mood" can be better viewed as blocking the emotions that exist. Neither chemical depression nor chemical euphoria are emotions, per se. There is a difference between the pain produced when a drug is injected and anger that the pain evokes.

5. The spread of the feeling of emotion from the emotion sites does not follow neurological or vascular pathways. Instead the spread is radial, extending and expanding in all directions at once. And it is rapid. This movement crosses numerous tissue change barriers, any or all of which would severely impede the rapid transference of any biochemical.

All of this suggests that while biochemistry is certainly involved with the reactions to emotions, emotion itself is not biochemical in nature.

> *There is more than enough evidence to suggest that emotion is far more than either a thought process or a biological process, and that it is something other than the child of both. Emotion appears to be an autonomous entity, with effects on both the mental and the physical.*

1 Emotion is:
  a. A byproduct of the body's biochemistry.
  b. A function of the limbic system.
  c. A subset of the brain process.
  d. Autonomous.

2. Emotion occurs:
  a. In the brain.
  b. As a result of neural messages.
  c. In the torso.
  d. Inside the organs.

3. Stress affects people:
  a. Differently because of genetic differences.
  b. Differently because of childhood training.
  c. According to their personal emotions.
  d. According to which emotion is repressed.

4. Which of these statements is (are) correct
  a. The expression of emotion occurs in specific body regions.
  b. The expression of emotion occurs in the hands and feet.
  a. The experience of emotion occurs in specific body regions.
  b. The experience of emotion occurs in the hands and feet.

5. Mood elevators:
  a. Create new emotions.
  b. Block emotional experience.
  c. Subdue the physical response to emotion.
  d. Transform poor emotions into better ones.

CHAPTER 7

FIELD-LIKE EFFECTS OF EMOTION

Curiously, better explanations for many of the properties and effects of emotion can be found in physics than can be found in either biology or psychology. When it is compared and examined from the perspective of physics, emotion is seen to have all the characteristics of a field in physics, being similar in nature to sound fields, radiant energy fields, fields of moving charges such as magnetism and electrostatics and the circulating energy fields that are the core of weather systems.

OBSERVATIONS OF FIELD-LIKE EFFECTS IN EMOTION

Most people, at one time or another, have experienced emotions that seemed to originate in another person, or persons and not in themselves. Emotions they experience almost, but not quite, as if their own.

Why are many people able to "sense" or "feel" another person's emotions without visual or audible clues? How does mass hysteria (mass emotion) sweep through crowds of otherwise normal, rational people? Why do people report feeling profound love when in the presence of a spiritual guru?

FEELING ANOTHER PERSON'S EMOTION The feeling of being caught in the experience of another's emotion is fairly common. The explanation that our own, subconscious, emotion was triggered by unwittingly observing some subtle body language or action of the other person may be true part of the time but certainly not all. Sometimes we approach someone from the rear where we can see nothing of the person's actions and suddenly we feel anger, or some other emotion. Or we may be involved with a conversation at our table in a restaurant and become aware of an unexplainable melting sensation in our heart only to discover a previously unobserved couple, wildly in love, at the next table. For people who have become emotionally open and receptive, these experiences may be fairly common.

It is not uncommon to enter a room where an emotion is sensed that seems to pervade the room, sensed long before any cognition of events in the room takes place: indeed, long before any events began to take place. Statements such as, "The fear was so thick you could cut it with a knife" or, "The room was full of fear" are common in these situations. These statements imply that the observer felt the emotion and recognized what it was *but was not caught up in it*, that is, felt the fear but was not afraid. The impersonal fear was not produced internally even though it was sensed internally. This situation is a much different one than if the observer had been subconsciously triggered by frightening actions or objects and had become personally afraid. *In that case, the observer would have said, "I was afraid" instead of, "The room was full of fear."*

THE PRESENCE OF A SPIRITUAL GURU The effect of true spiritual gurus on those who draw near them is a much grandeur form of experiencing another person's emotion. While emotions can be evoked because of expectation, something like the excitement of finally seeing the parade come around the corner, the effect of the spiritual Guru appears to be much more than this. There are many former disbelievers who report that they were "overwhelmed by something profound" when in the presence of the guru. On being questioned, those having had that experience usually describe it in terms of deep emotion, emotions that we call "heart emotions"; bliss, floods of love, joy, or ecstasy. Sometimes the receivers of these emotions report that initially they felt a great pain or wrenching in the heart area followed by the heart emotion. Often these experiences happen without even a word or a glance from the guru, simply being in the guru's presence is enough. (This is evidently the kind of effect that Jesus produced on those nearby, during his latter years.)

GROUP MEDITATION This is another instance where profound emotion that is not self generated can be experienced. And it is one where the possibility of visible or other clues is extremely unlikely. In meditation the meditators sit in silence, usually with their eyes closed. At times, profound love can sweep through the group, often bringing silent tears of joy or sadness to many. At other times a feeling of deep peacefulness (which is an emotion) is experienced throughout the room. These emotions are often experienced by others, immediately upon entering the room.

MASS HYSTERIA Frequently people report being swept up in the feeling of the moment and find themselves doing things that they are later quite unable to explain or understand. This effect has usually been dismissed with the notion that masses of humans can suddenly be triggered into temporary insanity simply by observing others in a state of panic or rage. This idea often leads to the conclusion that civilization is but a thin veneer, likely to be cracked at any time *merely by observing uncivilized behavior in others*. This conclusion is certainly questionable, to say the least. This notion is not accepted by any who believe that humans have either an innate drive, or a preborn drive towards goodness and wholeness. Mass hysteria is clearly outside of the scope of ordinary explanation, but certainly fits the concept of an emotional field, having effects capable of crossing space, much better than the notion that observing hysterical actions produce hysterical actions in the observer.

Sometimes pheromones (biochemicals produced by insects for use as sexual attractants) being dissipated through the air have been suggested as cause for this phenomenon but it occurs too rapidly for pheromones or other biochemical agents to be the cause. There are no biological mechanisms known that can shoot agents into the air that rapidly, nor could such chemicals cross long distances, especially if it were windy. And, there are no receptors in the body to receive and/or internalize such agents rapidly. In addition, pheromones are only known to be associated with sexual attraction, particularly in lower order insect and animal life. They are not known to be involved with emotions such as anger, fear, love or confidence.

The possibility of biological agents being involved with the experience of the guru is even less likely than the phenomena that occurs between two individuals. The quantity of these agents that would be required to create this effect, and to do it over such a wide area, would have to be extremely large and, again, none are known to exist.

This characteristic of emotion, the ability of emotion to cross the space between one person and another is impossible to explain from either the biochemical or mental models. However, the phenomena are those one finds in radiating fields such as sound fields or radio fields. If each person has a field of emotion in and around him or herself, the transference of emotion would be expected, since a vibration occurring in one field would resonate in nearby fields and the experience would be shared by all.

THE MENTAL MODEL OF EMOTION

The central tenet in this model is that emotion is the result of, or a byproduct of, mental or thought processes. The hard core of this school assumes that when unpleasant emotions occur, correcting the thought process will cause the disagreeable emotions to vanish. At best, this is not an easy concept to put into practice.

But does thinking actually produce emotion? - Always? Or just sometimes? Is emotion a sub-class or derivative of thought? Do the two experiences, thought and emotion, occur in the same location, act the same, feel the same? If emotions are just a sub-class of thought why can't we control our emotions with our thoughts?

THE DIFFERENCES BETWEEN THOUGHTS AND EMOTIONS

LOCATION All thinking occurs inside the brain but all emotion is experienced outside the brain. This seems to be the same for all people. Unemotional people who have deeply repressed their emotions sometimes presume that emotion is in their heads because that is where they think about emotion, or about emotionally charged events; but this experience is not emotion, it is the experience of *thinking* and occurs this way when the actual experience of *emotion* is repressed.

SOMATIC AFFECT The actual experience of emotion occurs in the torso. Interestingly enough, many of the more "primitive" or "less advanced" cultures have accepted the idea of a separate *emotional self* or *lower self* contained in the abdomen. The concept of a *visceral brain* being involved with emotion is not new. The Sufis, who were noted for their observations on psychology, refer to a center just below the navel, as being the seat of the *commanding self* that normally is in control of the emotions. Gurdjieff, who drew from a vast array of Eastern doctrines proposed the existence of a separate *emotional brain*, directing much of our actions from an abdominal location. Considering the tremendous effect emotion has on our lives this was not an unreasonable conclusion.

SPECIFIC SITES OF EMOTION Not only does the experience of emotion occur outside of the brain, in the torso, but it occurs in one of five specific locations, or emotion regions in the torso. The experiences of love and sadness are felt at the heart, experiences of anger and common fear at the solar plexus, experiences of confidence and guilt at the navel region, the experience of sexualness at the pubic region and the experience of mortal fear at the perineum. None of the various emotions are experienced inside the brain. There may be thoughts associated with the emotions but that is not the same thing as the emotion itself. And emotions often occur without associated thoughts.

The locations for the two experiences, emotion and thought, are mutually exclusive. If emotions were just a type of thought we would expect them to be experienced in the brain.

TYPE OF EXPERIENCE **(A)**. The experience of thought is quite different from the experience of emotion; we do not "feel" thoughts, but we do "feel" emotions. **(B)** And while there is only one experience of thought (unless it is tinged with a concurrent emotional experience) there are a variety of experiences of emotion. In spite of their similarities, the sensory experiences of emotion vary greatly from emotion to emotion. The feeling of love is quite different from the feeling of guilt and each of these feelings is quite different from the feelings of fear or sexuality or confidence.

CONTROL We can think a thought into existence but we cannot think an emotion into existence. About all that can be called up are thoughts about emotion (which is not the experience of emotion) unless there is a great pool of a particular emotion lurking just below the surface. Thinking about the incident that caused this pool of unresolved (suppressed, unfinished) emotion may activate the emotion, causing it to flower. In other words, the only time we can "think" an emotion into existence is when it is already there. Therefore, we did not think it into existence, the thought just brought it to the surface.

We can think and rethink a particular thought over and over as often as we try and the thought does not change in quality or experience. This is not true of the experience of emotion, we cannot try to re-experience an emotion again and again without losing it, eventually it just wears out. If emotions were end products of thought one should be able to call up any emotion at will and have the experience of it, over and over, just as we can with a thought.

Conversely, we **can** stop thinking a thought without much difficulty but we **cannot** stop an emotion by not thinking about it. Nor can we stop it by trying to think it out of existence. The emotion continues to intrude, not only in the form of remembering the scenario that originally caused it, but by coloring all our thoughts of other issues, as well. Statements such as "I got up on the wrong side of the bed" or "I'm in a foul mood" are common. When these conditions occur everything that happens to us will be colored by that festering emotion. It often seems as if the emotion actively hunts for new reasons to exist, as if it had a "mind of its own". It is only necessary to try turning off one of these activated emotions by thinking it "off" in order to grasp the significance of this statement.

It is quite clear that emotion overrides thought. This is something that could not happen if emotions were simply the end products of a thought stream or if thoughts were dominant over emotion.

The operation of a brain whose function and output (thoughts) are altered by emotion is much the same as that of a computer whose function and output (data) are altered when swept by an extraneous magnetic or electrical field from an outside source.

Emotion acts exactly like an autonomous, changeable field, generated at some point in the body (one of the four loci referenced above - Heart, Solar Plexus, Navel and Pubic), sweeping across the brain, controlling brain output until the emotion ceases.

Figure 5 Field Effects

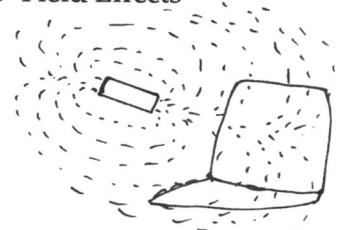

Magnetic Field
Altering Computer Output

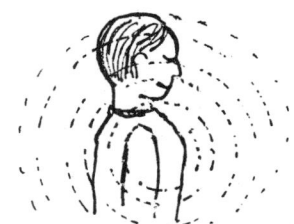

Emotion Altering
Brain Function and Output

The concept that there is a field of emotion that originates in the body and pervades the brain offers an explanation for two, at first glance, seemingly different conditions: rational thought and confusion.

RATIONAL THOUGHT.

But is rational thought really rational? The degree to which emotions control our thoughts is clearly shown when we examine the "rational" thought process. Rational thought is usually defined as being coherent and logical according to the information available. But that definition fails to account for the wide variances in the rational thoughts of different people in the same situation.

Supposedly, rational thought is devoid of emotional content. But is this ever possible? At one time or another, most of us have had the experience of thinking a series of thoughts that seemed completely rational given the facts of the situation and then having the entire chain of "rational" thought crumble as our emotion changed. *The facts as we saw them had not changed, but our rational thought sequence had.*

A person in the grip of anger often undertakes actions that seem totally logical (to them) at the time only to find that they cannot support that rationality when they are in a different emotional state. ("I don't know what got into me"). Or a person will take actions while in a state of fear that they simply cannot understand, or explain as being rational, when they are no longer in that fear state.

Two people, one in a state of love and the other in a state of anger can walk down the street side by side and perceive the identical event happening and put entirely different "rational" meanings to it. When their emotional states are different their conclusions and judgments will be poles apart.

"Rational" seems not to have as much to do with objective reality as it does with consistency. Since the basis for our thoughts always changes as our emotions change, it would be more accurate to define rationality by its emotion, by the prevailing emotion being experienced at the time. If we were to say, "rational as while experiencing love" or, "rational as when a state of anger", we would be much closer to the truth of it.

If it is to be realistic, rational thought must be defined by the emotional base upon which it rests, not only its tone but its consistency as well. *When the emotional base is constant, the thoughts will be ordered and coherent but the direction or tone of the thoughts will be governed by the emotion that is being experienced.* Here again, emotion appears to sweep the brain and alter its function. Now, if this concept is indeed valid, it would have to apply equally well to the process of confusion, or non-coherent fluctuating thought.

CONFUSION - OR CONFUSED THOUGHT?

When in a confused state we do not say that our thoughts are confused. Instead we say "I feel confused". Upon reflection, confused thought appears simply to be disorganized, nonrational thought. But why is it disorganized? Why has the thought process become fragmented, which it is in confusion? What prevents logic from ordering our thoughts?

The person in the confused state is usually aware of an unpleasant shifting mood or emotional state. Why does this happen? Are the unpleasant emotional feelings a reaction to the disturbed thinking process? That is, do we have unpleasant feelings because we are upset at our illogical thinking? Observing the facial expression and body language shifts when an obviously confused person is speaking presents quite a different picture.

The process occurs in three distinct steps. The facial or body language shifts occur first (signaling a change in emotion). This is followed by a pause and, finally, by a statement from an entirely different emotional perspective. *That perspective is indicative of the new emotion being experienced.* If the thoughts had changed first, we would have heard new statements **before** the facial expression and body language changed.

When the emotional shifts are too rapid for the person to follow, their thoughts cannot keep up, chains of thought falter and break and confused thinking results. The person in the confused state will usually say, "I feel confused". (It is rather telling that when people are in this state they do not say, "I think confused".)

I stumbled onto the nature of confusion many years ago while doing SHEN Physioemotional Release Therapy with an older woman who was troubled with a lot of buried emotion. While working in the region between the solar plexus and the navel, I was suddenly swept with the feeling of confusion. I recall being quite startled, wondering why I felt confused because my thoughts were not vacillating. My thought train was secure and remained so (except for being puzzled by the feeling of confusion). I really hadn't been thinking about anything much, just waiting for the flows to go through. I checked through my procedures to see if I was doing something wrong but I wasn't, so that wasn't causing my confusion. I just felt confused. Finally it tapered off and the session ended. But I remained puzzled. And I remained puzzled until the next time I worked with the woman.

As I worked in the same body region as before, the feeling of confusion swept over me again, and then I got it! **I was picking up and feeling the release of a jumble of her emotions!** *As I recall, she later confirmed that she couldn't sort out the emotions she was feeling at the time, they were too quick and random.*

Thought *patterns* change when and only when emotion shifts. Confusion is the result of rapid emotional shifts; the emotions surfacing one after another carry the thought stream in rapidly changing directions. The structure of the thought train is altered by the emotion of the moment, so much so that often a thought sequence vanishes in the middle of a sentence, leaving it to waver off in the face of the next emotion.

CONSISTENCY OF THOUGHT.

When the emotion being experienced is constant, logically ordered thinking with a tone matching the emotion being experienced results. This is *rational thought*. But when the emotions vary rapidly, confused and illogically ordered thinking, or *confused thought* results. When our emotional state is stable, our thinking is stable. The consistency of thought is governed by the constancy of the emotion being experienced while the tone or mood of thought is determined by the specific emotion being experienced.

Thus, both rational thought and confused thought appear to be the results of a changeable emotional field sweeping through the brain and altering its function, precisely as an extraneous electrostatic field alters the function of a computer "brain".

THE BIOCHEMICAL MODEL OF EMOTION

There is a considerable body of published work that attempts to define or understand emotion through an understanding of body chemistry where emotions are supposedly the byproducts of biochemical reactions. In this model the sensations we experience as (think are) emotions are merely the results of certain *as yet undiscovered* secretions that have been released into the bloodstream and body tissue. The usual diagram from this perspective is: external cause - is observed by the sensory organs and - assimilated and processed by the brain which - sends neurological messages to - the muscles, glands and organs - stimulating them into action - incidentally producing the biophysiological sensations which are called - *emotions*. But in order to reach this conclusion time and its relation to cause and effect must be overlooked because the experience of emotions occurs much faster than the biochemicals could move through the body. When the sequence is examined closely, emotion appears to affect the body in the same way that it affects the brain, as a field sweeping through tissue and altering certain responses.

On a recent PBS Television show on emotions, a biochemist remarked, "We have isolated the chemical that produces love". However, after a brief explanation of how this chemical would produce the emotion "love" in the body, he added, "Of course we can't produce the **mystical** experience of love". This is precisely where biochemical research into the nature of emotion always fails. It fails because the core experience of emotion is not a biological one but a mystical or metaphysical one.

CHEMISTRY, EMOTION AND THE BRAIN:

It is true that certain chemicals, mostly drugs of various legalities, can effect mood, but this is not the same as producing an emotion. Nor are the chemicals in these drugs the biochemicals involved in the physiological or biological reaction to emotion. Without going into considerable detail we see that elevating or depressing overall mood is not the same as inducing an emotion.

It might be more accurate to say that drugs block or alter the **perception** of emotion or block the **suppression** of emotion. A mood elevator blocks the brain's perception of the sadness or anger being repressed that caused the depression. "Anti-depressant" drugs are precisely named - they are not called "joy pills" because they do not produce joy. They merely block the perception of the depressed (repressed) emotions of sadness, anger or other emotions.

There is no question that chemicals can make us feel good or bad. Even the lack of certain dietary chemicals will produce sensations that can approximate emotions, although they cannot precisely duplicate them. Lack of either calcium or magnesium will produce an experience very much like anxiety. Those who have experienced both emotional anxiety and calcium/magnesium deficiency, and have paid attention to the nuances, know that there is a difference. Perhaps one condition should be called *emotional anxiety* and the other *chemical anxiety*.

With some emotions there is no connection between the locations of the emotional experience and the locations of their associated biochemical actions. With others there is no immediate, associated biological effect at all.

1. The feeling of sexual arousal (emotion) is experienced just above the pubic bone. It is true that this particular emotion site is close to the ovaries and the uterus which produce hormones and other secretions in the woman. But a man also experiences sexual *emotion* at this site however a man does not have sexual *glands* at this site.

2. Emotions of confidence, worthiness, achievement, unworthiness, guilt, adequacy and inadequacy are experienced at the emotion site just below the navel. There are no glands or organs near this site to supply the necessary chemistry to account for the experience of these emotions. Neither are there organs or glands in that location that are able to utilize any special biochemistry.

THE "FIGHT OR FLIGHT RESPONSE".
This response is often brought up as an example to show that emotion is the result of a shift in the body's biochemistry. It is explained that what we experience as fear is the sensation of epinephrine (adrenaline) being released into the bloodstream from the adrenals. (When the adrenal glands, which are located close to the spine at the solar plexus, are stimulated by fear the medullas of the adrenals release extra amounts of epinephrine into the bloodstream. Epinephrine is necessary to convert large amounts of glycogen, which is stored in the liver, into pyruvate, which supports severe and prolonged muscular exertion.) A closer look at the entire process shows that this explanation is doubtful at best.

According to the usual theory, secondary effects of epinephrine are constriction of the blood vessels in the gut and kidney and inhibition of the secretory activities in the gastrointestinal tract. Supposedly, restricting gut blood flow makes the blood available to the muscles in the limbs. **But at the same time the blood vessels in the gut et al. are being *constricted*, blood vessels in the extremities become *dilated and relaxed*.** Both, according to the usual theory, *by the same epinephrine*.

Obviously, this is a major contradiction. How can the epinephrine cause smooth muscle in some blood vessels to contract and smooth muscle in other vessels to dilate? To explain this dichotomy, it is proposed that there are two types of membrane receptors (alpha or beta) in the muscle cells. Supposedly smooth muscle tissue with the alpha receptor would relax when influenced by epinephrine and tissue with the beta receptor would contract. In addition to the fact that these receptors have never been located, there are other serious shortcomings to this model.

EXAMINING THE EXPERIENCE OF FEAR.

1. *The experience, or feeling, of fear begins at the solar plexus and **expands outward in all directions***. However the blood supply does not radiate outward from that center. The major arteries (carriers of epinephrine and the various biochemical intermediaries) follow the spine. If epinephrine were responsible for the experience of fear, the pattern of expanding fear should move up and down the spine, but it doesn't, it expands outward in a circle.

2. It is not possible for epinephrine to migrate in the radial pattern that fear takes. It cannot because it would have to pass through and cross many different and varied tissues which would cause chemical reactions that would alter or destroy the epinephrine before it had passed the first barrier. Epinephrine could not possibly be the cause of the expanding disc of fear.

3. Sometimes when faced with fear, instead of being mobilized into action as might be expected because of the abundance of pyruvate in the bloodstream, the physical body freezes and becomes immobilized. This is the reverse of what one would expect if epinephrine were the cause of the fear experience. Supposedly more epinephrine would produce greater fear and this should result in more action, not less.

4. In order to explain why different people react differently in the face of the same fear provoking stimulus (some run, some fight, others freeze), it is proposed that perhaps variable ratios of epinephrine and norepinephrine (a cousin with similar but slightly different effects) are secreted by different individuals. This has not been demonstrated.

5. Interestingly enough, nicotine, histamine, reserpine, acetylcholne, morphine, ether, low blood sugar, insulin and exercise all stimulate the release of epinephrine but *do not cause cause the experience of fear.*

6. Anger stimulates the adrenal medulla, exactly as fear does, to release epinephrine and, even though the two are closely related, the experience of anger is quite different from the experience of fear. Two different emotions would not likely be produced by the same chemical.

THE ENERGY FIELD MODEL OF THE FIGHT OR FLIGHT RESPONSE

1. Fear radiates outward from its point of origin at the solar plexus.
2. In order to halt the unpleasant experience of fear, the body contracts around the center of the fear (the solar plexus/diaphragm).
3. Tension affects all muscle tissue including smooth muscle tissue.
4. Tension around the solar plexus limits capillary perfusion through the digestive organs and the transverse colon.
5. But the arms and legs are not affected because they are far from that center.
6. The cold feeling sometimes experienced at the pit of the stomach is the result of the area being under the greatest tension. It is cold because of reduced blood flow.
7. The contraction of fear can become so intense that it can produce a reaction across the entire body. When it does, the entire body freezes, as legs and arms are immobilized because of the tension.
8. On occasion the contraction against fear is so great that, as it squeezes the transverse colon, defecation occurs.

The pattern of emotion radiating outward from a point is the same motion found in fields in physics. This pattern is found in sound fields, electromagnetic radiation and the ripples from a stone cast into a stream.

WHICH CAME FIRST? EMOTION OR BIOCHEMICAL CHANGE.

This is not to say that biochemistry is not involved with the emotions at all. But "being involved with" and "being a result of" are very different things.

*If emotions are not the **result** of biochemistry, could they be the **cause** of biochemical change? If emotions are something other than biochemistry, which is doing the acting and which is reacting? Which begins the process, the emotion or the chemical change? Do changes in the body's biochemistry produce the new emotion or could the emerging emotion be causing the change in the body's biochemistry? These questions have complex answers. However, we can at least begin to unravel them.*

In the example of fear and epinephrine, it is difficult to imagine how the chemical action could have taken place before the fear was experienced. *If we stop to think about it, we can see that the emotion must precede the biochemical action or else there would be no reason for the chemical action to begin.*

Then we must ask, "Would the fear, which is experienced exactly at the adrenals, alert the brain to signal the adrenals to release adrenaline, an unlikely sequence - *or does the fear directly cause the release of adrenaline by bathing the adrenals in the emotion?"* If so, this effect would be identical to the effect of a field shift affecting the brain, as detailed earlier.*

THE FIELD THEORY OF EMOTION

Emotion gives every evidence of being, not just "emotion", or even many "emotions", but an **emotional field**, one that permeates and affects the entire human body as well as the mind.

Emotion is a metaphysical (nonbiological) experience usually paralleled by biological, or physical responses and by mental or psychological processes. Emotions are produced and experienced in a **physioemotional field** which behaves as other fields in physics behave. The state or condition of this field affects the glands and organs, including the brain, whose function is modified or distorted by the emotions.

Since it is a field, it is possible for the experience of an individual emotion to be transmitted from one person's field to another. Because of this, one person's field can be altered by specific interjections of another person's field. (This process can be used to treat psychosomatic disorders, and to accelerate and end anxiety and depression.)

1. Thought does not control emotion because we cannot start or stop an emotion by thinking of it or about it. Emotion appears to predominate over thought.

2. The state or condition of the emotional field affects brain function, causing our thoughts to be either **rational** (consistent) or **confused** (random). *We can think rationally only in accord with the particular emotion being experienced at the moment.* In a state of confusion, it is the shifting emotional base that shifts the tone of our thoughts.

3. Because it is a field, emotion can be transmitted through space and directly experienced by those near the originator of the emotion.

4. Suppressed emotion can be evoked and released from one persons emotion centers by passing the energy from another person's hands through those emotion centers.

5. The glands and organs located in the vicinity of each emotion center are directly affected by the emotion being produced (and/or suppressed) by that center through contractile tensions developed in the body to repress the feeling of emotion.

1. Why are some people able to "feel" another person's emotions without visual or aural clues?

2. Which is true:
   a. Thoughts control emotions.
   b. Emotions control thoughts.

3. Pheromones are byproducts of emotion.
   T.
   F.

4. Which is (are) true:
   a. Fear is a result of Epinephrine.
   b. Fear is a byproduct of Epinephrine.
   c. Neither.
   d. Both.

5. We can stop emotion if we can stop thinking about it long enough.
   T.
   F.

CHAPTER 8

PHYSICS OF THE PHYSIOEMOTIONAL FIELD

THE QUESTION OF EVIDENCE

A transducer[25] is needed in order to measure the physioemotional field. Unfortunately however, none has yet been discovered. But although the field is not measurable in the way that electricity can be measured, there is considerable empirical evidence to show that the field exists and some information as to its quality and state as well. (Actually, the body is a transducer of sorts since body temperature shifts occur when the field through the body is increased.)

HAND SENSATIONS. It is relatively easy for most people to sense the field. Bringing the palm of one hand close to another person's, or close to your other hand, lets you detect various subtle sensations, especially in the palm.[26] These sensations are usually perceived as changes in temperature (most often heat, although some perceive it as coolness), tingles, prickles, "electricity" (the sensation of light static), pressure or "magnetism". The sensations behave as would be expected, the closer to the subject the greater the sensation.

1. In addition, these sensations are observed to change in intensity and in quality concurrent with, or slightly after, physiological changes are observed in persons receiving SHEN Therapy. This is usually noted as an increase in heat and usually occurs immediately following an episode of REM, a myoclonic jerk or a sudden breath change.

2. The sensations are usually different when the hand is over an area of physical pain, inflammation, tension and/or when release of emotion occurs when the hand is over an emotion region. The sensations picked up over an area of pain do not feel the same as the ones over a center that is releasing emotion. (Not all practitioners experience every type of sensory difference, however there is a high level of consistency.)

3. Polar Differences. There appears to be a polar difference between the two hands as one appears to emit energy and the other to receive it. (This polar difference is consistent with other fields in physics.) This polarity is confirmed by a particular sequence of events. Usually, when doing a flow through a person, a sensation of pressure builds in one hand, the **sending hand** for a time until it suddenly disappears. Immediately after this, a physiological reaction occurs in the patient/client and this, in turn, is followed by a noticeable increase in sensation in the second, the **receiving hand**. These sensations do not always occur but when they do they always start and finish in the same hands.

---

[25] A transducer is a device which converts one kind of energy to another. A phonograph cartridge converts motion to electrical energy and a solar cell converts light to electricity. Transducers are necessary in order to measure anything. Without them there would be no meters of any sort. *Actually, the hand is a transducer of sorts, since it is able to detect quantitative differences in the field.*

[26] The same effect occurs when the hands are near certain crystalline structures, especially quartz.

Several experiments were undertaken to try to establish if body heat, infra-red radiation, a low potential DC electrical field or a weak magnetic field were the cause of the phenomena.

Measurement of temperature changes
Since the changes noted in the palms are usually perceived as changes in heat, it was decided to take temperature measurements at the palm of the receiving hand to see if there was an actual change in temperature.

Figure 6
Temperature
Measurement

Probe connected
to receiving hand

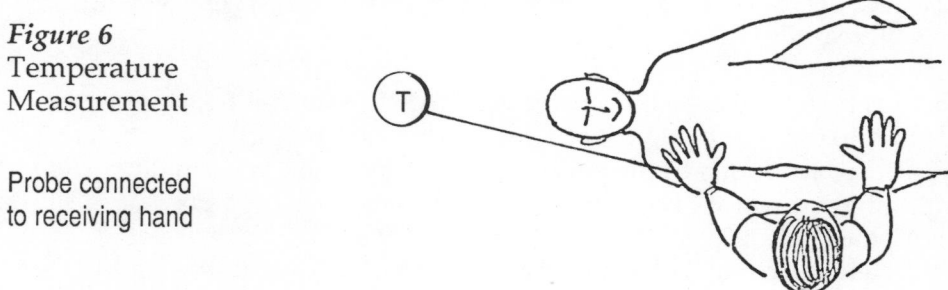

This experiment confirmed that the sensation was not imaginary and that there is an increase in heat coincident with the increase in sensory experience. However the experiment did not determine if heat was being radiated directly from one hand to the other or whether it was caused by the body heat of the other person.

The measurements were then re-taken with the hands separated from the body by three inch foam cushions. It took longer for the flows to move through the greater distance, but they did and the physiological effects noted were the same. This experiment established that it was not the other person's body heat that caused the effect. (Note that the sending hand is under the body and the receiving hand is on top.)

Figure 7
Temperature
Measurements
Through
Insulation

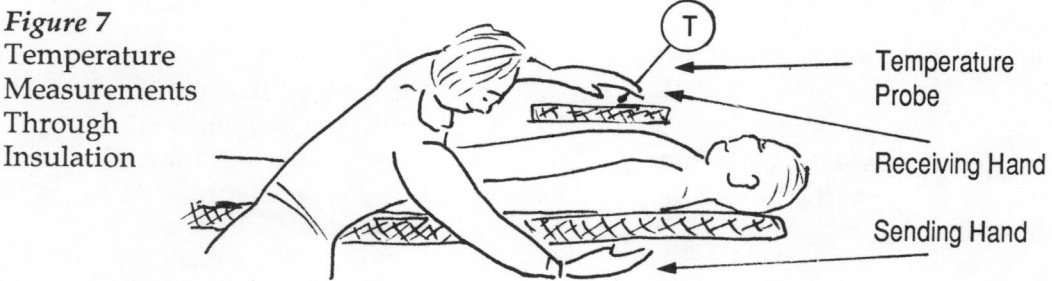

Temperature
Probe

Receiving Hand

Sending Hand

Now, this experiment clearly showed that a transference of *something* occurred, but of what? It was not likely that it was caused by actual heat because the foam pillows were insulators. Could some other effect be transferred from one hand to the other that would cause a change in capillary perfusion? (As mentioned earlier, an increase of heat in the skin requires an increase in capillary perfusion.) To definitely establish whether the operant was heat transfer or some other medium, the experiment was modified to include three more temperature gauges[27], all of which were separated by foam insulators.

---

[27] Temperatures were measured with two J&J Model T-68's and a J&J Digital Integrator Model D-200.

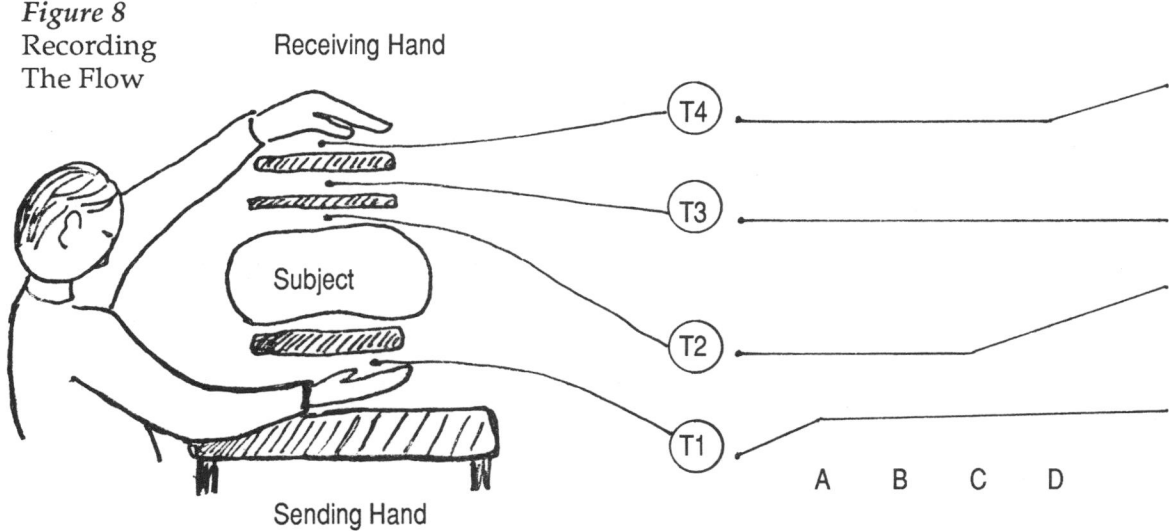

Figure 8
Recording
The Flow

Receiving Hand

T4

T3

Subject

T2

T1

A B C D

Sending Hand

This experiment proved quite interesting. The first effect noted was that the temperature gauge connected to the sending hand elevated several degrees in a linear fashion while the others showed no appreciable change. (Some of this initial increase was because the sending hand was between two 3" foam insulators.) After several minutes a distinct sequence of events took place. (A) At this point the rate of temperature rise in the sending hand leveled to almost flat. (B) About fifteen seconds later the subject released a mild myoclonic jerk and breath rate slowed. (C) Ten seconds later, the temperature reading at the subject's stomach began to rise. (D) Finally, fifteen seconds after the temperature rise at her stomach, the temperature at the receiving hand began to rise rapidly, increasing nearly a degree before leveling out.

But the most exciting reading was from the third probe, between the two insulating cushions. *The reading on this gauge never changed, but remained constant throughout the experiment.* This proves conclusively that the field effect is some medium other than heat, or infrared radiation.

This experiment shows there is a definite transference of effect from the sending hand, through the subject's body, to the receiving hand. The experiment has been repeated several times with the same results.

OTHER EXPERIMENTS

RELAXATION EFFECT. A further experiment showed that the increase in the temperature of the subject's body was not just due to relaxation. (When a person relaxes deeply their skin temperature usually goes up.) Identical temperature sensors were placed on the subject's body at: the solar plexus, the heart, the throat and between the navel and solar plexus. The subject was covered with a one inch sheet of foam insulation and successive SHEN flows were performed. These started from the root, passed through the spine and then exited out: (1) the solar plexus, (2) the heart and (3) the throat. (The gauge between the navel and solar plexus was the control, no flows were done through it.)

Figure 9 Flows At Successive Sites

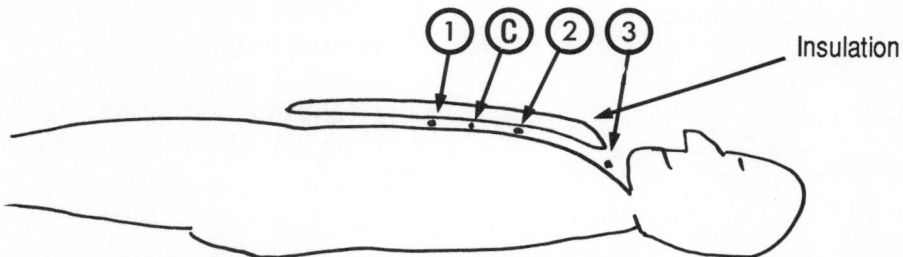

As each flow was performed in turn, the temperature at the associated gauge rose perceptibly only to fall back as the flow was halted and the next flow began. The control gauge, while it rose slightly in the beginning as the subject relaxed, did no more than that, it never showed the sharp rise that the other gauges did when flows were done through their sites.

A surprising thing happened during the heart flow. The subject gave a large myoclonic jerk and her breath rate dropped sharply. Immediately all the temperature gauges began rapidly dropping except the one at the heart *which rose dramatically to end with the highest reading of all*. Evidently blood volume dropped as her breath rate dropped (which would be expected). The fact that the skin temperature at the heart rose the way it did indicates that the flow of energy caused the capillaries in that region to open more than usual.

VOLTAGE AND MAGNETIC MEASUREMENTS. 1. A micro-voltmeter[28] connected between the sending and receiving hands indicates a zero potential, showing that the physio-emotional field is not likely to be a DC field. (It has been suggested that the field may be some as yet undetected high frequency field. This is possible but not likely; in order to generate a high frequency alternating field, there would have to be a source of activity in the body which would alternate at that high frequency as well as produce electricity.)

2. Since sensitive magnetic coils do not pick up evidence of a magnetic field either, it is not likely that the field is magnetic.

POLAR EFFECTS OF THE FIELD. Early in the development of SHEN it was discovered that if the therapist places his or her right hand on the patient's right hip and their left hand on the patient's right shoulder, in a short time the person begins to relax, may fall asleep, and later awakens refreshed. These effects are considered to be beneficial and healthy. *The flow between the therapist's hands was moving **upward** through the person's right side.*

Figure 10
Normal Flow

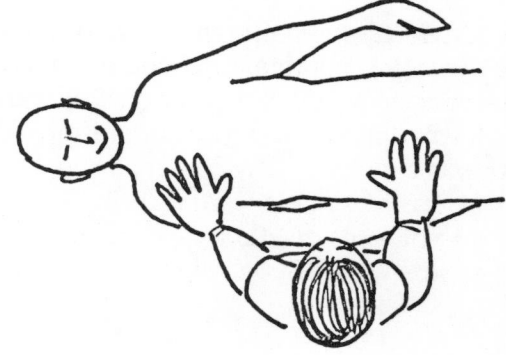

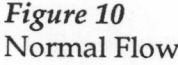
[28] Hickock Model LX-304

However, if the therapist reverses the order of their hands (left hand on the right hip and right hand on the right shoulder) a very different effect will occur. Soon, the patient's heart begins beating faster and, if the reversed flow continues long enough, causes discomfort, disorientation and, if done long enough, nausea. These are not healthy effects. (The flow was moving **downward** through the right side of the person's torso.) NOTE: This procedure is NOT normally performed during SHEN Therapy sessions.

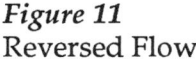
Figure 11
Reversed Flow

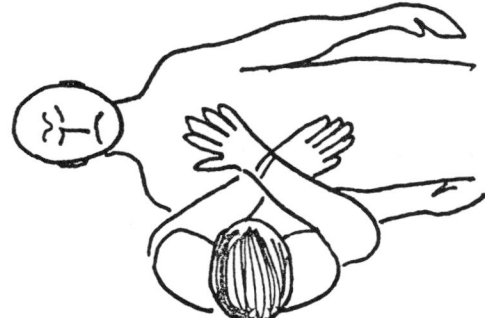

The conclusion was made that the flow direction that produces healthy effects would have to be the direction of normal flow through the body.

There is a second observation that supports this conclusion. It takes longer for the flow to move between the hands in the second example (Fig. 11) than in the first (Fig. 10). This is exactly what happens when two flows are in opposition. Flows in conjunction in confluent fields move swiftly, those in opposition take much longer, as well as causing turbulence in their flows.

ORGANIZATION AND PATTERN OF THE FLOWS

It seemed logical to assume, since the laws of apparent motion within these fields are common to all, that the same laws would apply to the physioemotional field as well. The observations shown above, plus an understanding of the rules of order in physics that relate to magnetism, electricity, weather currents and hydraulics, led to the determination of the field patterns that are shown next. The validity and accuracy of the patterns were established by the results of the clinical work that was based on those patterns.

*(It is common to refer to the physioemotional field as an **energy field**. Technically this is incorrect because in physics the word **energy** refers to work being done or to energy consumed. Coal has energy to heat water, food has energy to power the body. These types of energy are measured in calories or in BTU's. The physioemotional field is not an energy of this type.)*

The physioemotional field is not just an amorphous mass or cloud without order or direction, it has the same arrangement of circulating patterns found in the other fields. These patterns are similar in formation and function to magnetic fields or electrostatic fields. The patterns formed by iron filings that are sprinkled on a sheet of paper over the poles of a magnet are an example.

THE PERIPHERAL BODY FLOWS

Considerable experimenting showed that
the flow of the field through the right side
of the body moves in an **upward** direction,
from foot to shoulder and the flow through
the body's left side moves **downward**, from
shoulder to foot.

But the flows do not end at the shoulders
and feet. The laws of physics governing
field circulation require that the ends of the
flows connect to make complete circuits.
What happens can be seen when two
magnets are placed side by side.

Figure 12
Peripheral Flows

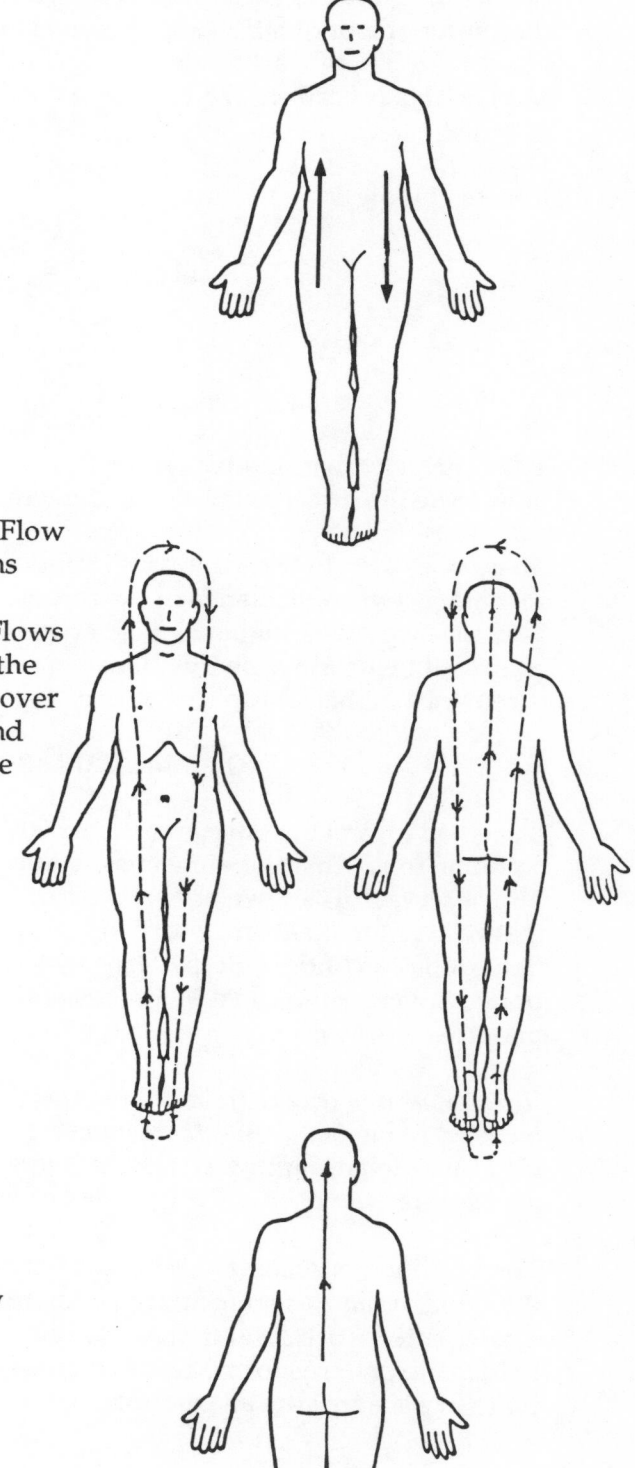

Figure 13
Magnetic Field
Connections

When two magnets
are placed side by
side with their
poles reversed the
flows connect like
this:

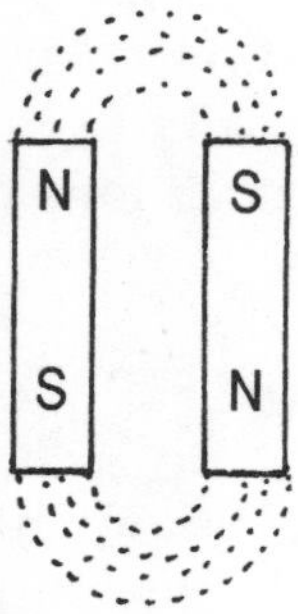

Figure 14
Peripheral Flow
Connections

The body Flows
connect in the
same way, over
the head and
between the
feet.

Figure 15 The Halo Effect

(When fully developed, the
head loop is sometimes
faintly visible. When it
is, it is called a **Halo**.)

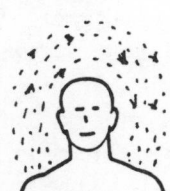

Figure 16
Spinal Flow

There is one other long flow in the body.
This is a concentrated flow that moves up
the spine from the perineum to the crown.

THE ARM/HAND FLOW.

The other major circulating flow moving through the body is in the arms. The flow exits from one hand and eventually returns to the other, just as it does in a magnet. (Remember, all circulating fields must return to their source, they can't just dissipate in space.)

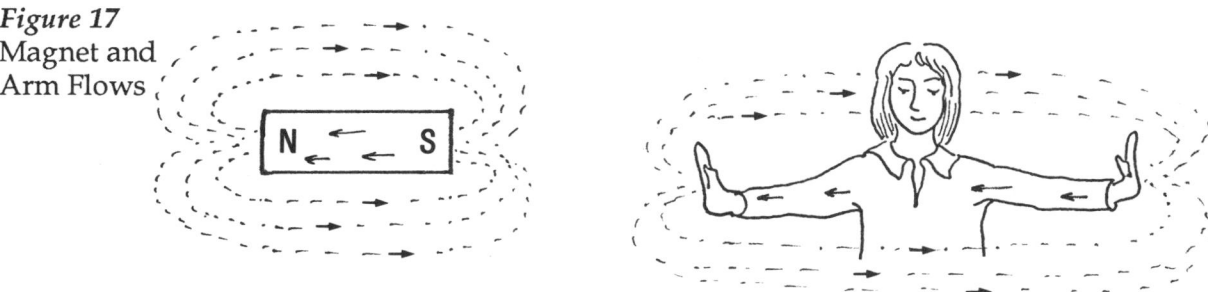

Figure 17
Magnet and
Arm Flows

With most people, the flow exits the right hand & comes back to the left.

Figure 18 Increasing the Flows
With either the magnet or the hand/arm flows, moving the ends closer together increases the effect as all of the lines of force merge and the field becomes concentrated. (This increases the effectiveness of the flow and explains why it is harder to get a flow to move through another person's body when your hands are farther apart.)

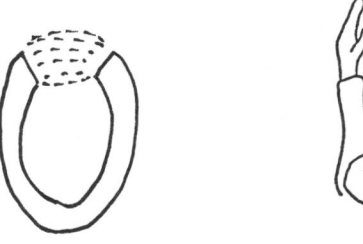
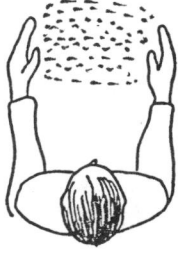

Figure 19 Peripheral, Arm and Spinal Flows

FILLING THE BODY

All of the body's tissue is permeated by the field. Single arrows were used in all the preceding drawings to indicate the direction of flow (movement) but it should be understood that the flows completely fill the portion of the body they travel through, not just the tiny lines indicated by the arrows.

NOTE: If you are using this handbook to learn how to do SHEN, turn to the next chapter, BASIC SHEN, as you have all the theory you need for the moment. You will be directed when to turn back to this section for the theory you will need later.

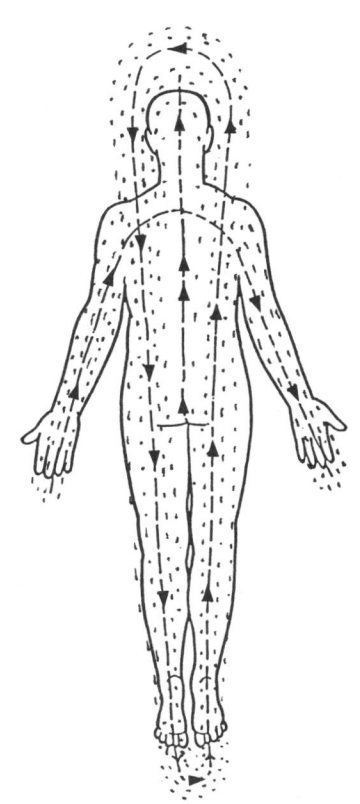

THE THREE PART PATTERN

The flow patterns of all fields in physics are composed of three parts an Inner part, an Outer part and a small Helical (rotary) part which separates the other two. All circulating fields have a small helix between the inner and outer portions.

The three parts are found in the movements that form clouds. The clouds form when a column of warm air rises, is cooled, and leaves water vapor in a visible cloud as the air spills back to the ground. This falling air forms into a doughnut shape surrounding the column of rising air.

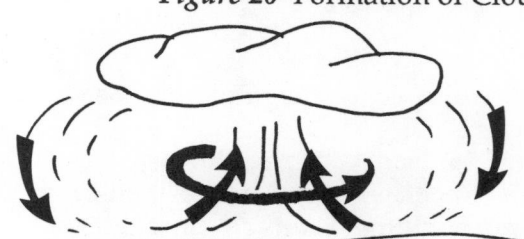

Figure 20 Formation of Clouds

When it reaches the ground, the air reheats and rises again in a continuous, circulating pattern. Besides the rising and falling components, a small rotary wind (helix) circles between the rising column and the falling doughnut.

You may have noticed this rotary wind effect if you have flown under a cloud in a small plane. As you approached the leading edge of the cloud the plane dipped sharply to the right and as it passed out from under the other side of the cloud it dipped sharply to the left. The dips were caused by crossing the rotary wind as it came first from the left and then from the right.

Figure 21
Passing Under
a Cloud

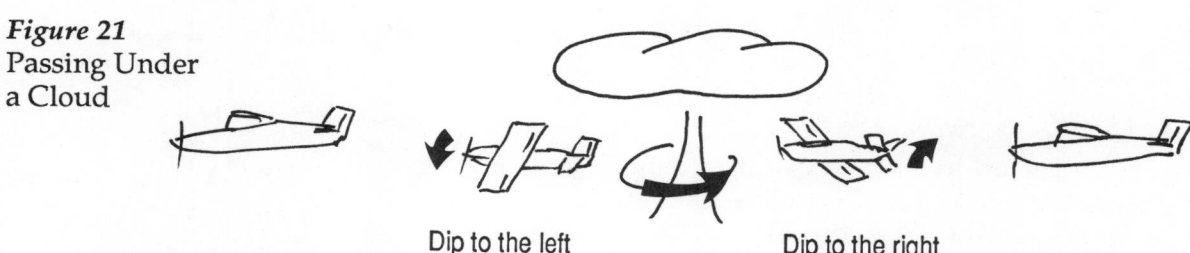

Dip to the left   Dip to the right

It is this same rotary wind that causes the sudden gust from the side as we face an approaching thunderstorm. And explains why there are opposing circular wind patterns around high and low pressure areas on weather maps.

ROTARY CURRENTS IN MAGNETS.

An **inner** flow moves through the magnet and exits out the North Pole, becoming the circular **outer** flow that returns to the magnet at the South Pole. (In the same way the inner flow of the physioemotional field moves through the body and then becomes the outer portion as it loops around the head.) Separating the two is the much smaller **helical** flow. The physioemotional field also has a helix.

Figure 22

Complete
Patterns
in Fields

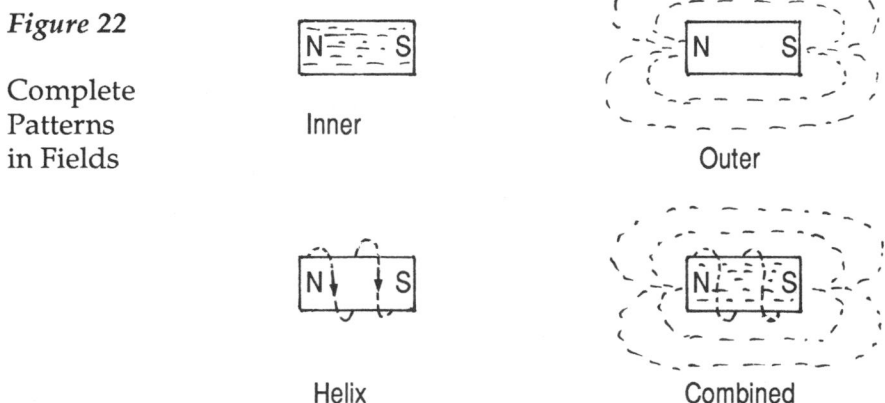

Inner

Outer

Helix

Combined

(You are familiar with helices, a screen door spring is a helix.)

Figure 23
Field Around the Arms

*The same rotating helix
occurs around the arms:*

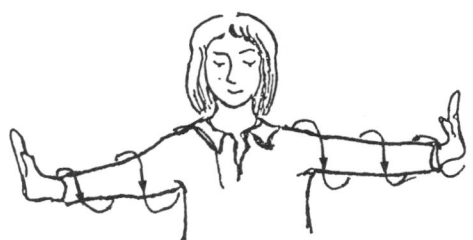

Figure 24 Matching the Helices

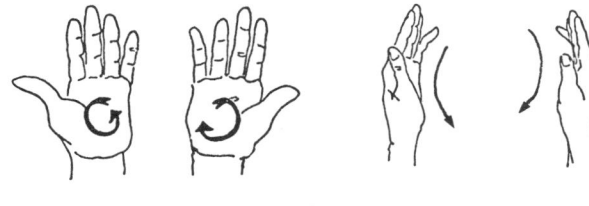

The ends of these helices appear to rotate in
opposite directions, at least when the hands
are held out, side by side. However, when
the hands are placed facing each other, they
are seen to line up.

Figure 25 The Body Helices

Circulating helices also surround the
peripheral flows through the two sides of
the body and are necessary to set the stage
for transference of emotion from one person
to another that was discussed earlier.

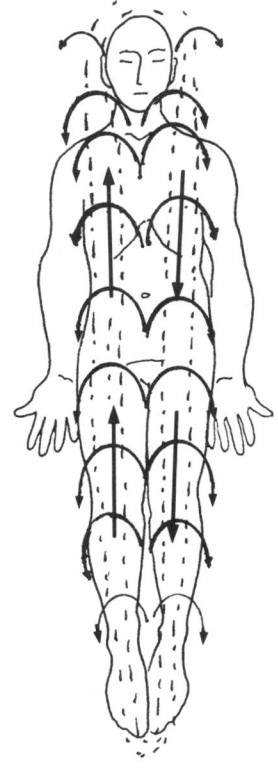

Figure 26 The Centers of Emotion

The peripheral flows form the
framework of the physioemotional
field. Within these flows,
centered along the spine,
are the centers of emotion.

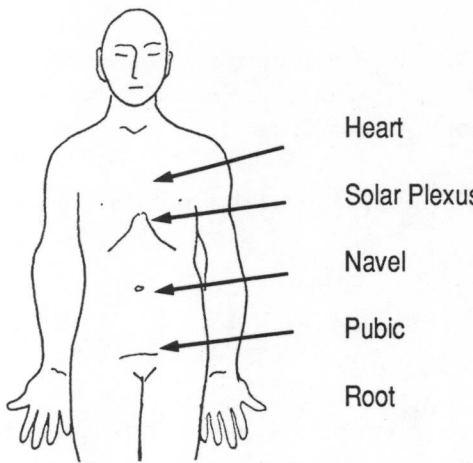

Heart

Solar Plexus

Navel

Pubic

Root

FIELD ACTION AT THE EMOTION CENTERS

The field behaves differently in the emotion centers than at other parts of the body. Something alters the field at these points to create the experience called *emotion*. While we are not certain of all the factors that might be involved in this, there is strong evidence to suggest that the effect is largely one of vibration. It seems that, under certain circumstances, the field begins to vibrate at those points and we feel the vibrations as emotions. There is evidence that supports this idea.

Several years ago, experiments were conducted by the author that linked sound vibrations with two of these centers, the heart and the solar plexus. Pure tones of different frequencies were sounded near subjects who were deeply relaxed during SHEN sessions. Later, the subjects reported that they "felt" these sounds at one or the other of these two centers. There was unanimous agreement as to which tones affected which centers. The one at the heart, in particular, produced a sensation similar to the emotions normally experienced there. While it cannot be entirely proven at this time, it does appear that, under the proper conditions, an **emotional vibration** occurs in the field at these points and that *there are distinct differences in vibratory frequencies at the different emotion centers.*[29]

Mixing the effects of vibration and flow is common in other fields in physics. Throwing a stone into a stream sends ripples vibrating in all directions, but the ripples do not disturb the downstream flow.

Expansion of the Vibrations. An interesting thing appears to happen to the vibrations in the field. As the vibrations build and increase, they expand and radiate outward from the emotion centers. This outward (frontward) movement is supported by the helices surrounding the main flows through the body (see Figure 25). *This expansion of the vibrating field is probably what allows us to sense, or feel, another person's emotion directly, as we step into their vibrations.*

---

[29] It is generally accepted that music (sound) affects the emotions. Most thinkers in this field ascribe the process involved to the auditory nervous system. (This is largely because no other possible pathway was perceived.) No one would deny the part of the auditory pathway in the process but, no one experiencing the difference in sensation of a powerful dance tune played through a stereo headset and the same tune played through loudspeakers would ever deny that there is a bodily component to the perception of sound.

As the field is moved outward at the emotion centers, it assumes the shape of an expanding bubble, just as sound waves do when coming from a speaker. There are two components to this motion, out the front and away from the center.

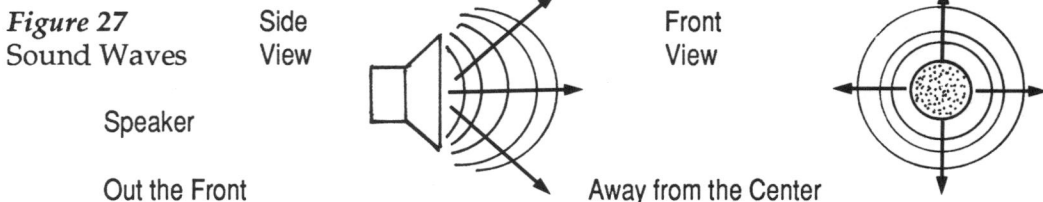

Figure 27
Sound Waves

Speaker

Out the Front

Side View

Front View

Away from the Center

The concept that emotion is largely in front of the body is supported by our experience of feeling another person's emotions. When we do feel them, we feel them far more intensely when in front of the person than when at the rear or sides.

Just as it was affected by the helices around the peripheral flow of energy through the body, the vibrating bubble is affected by the vertical motion of the peripheral flows. These two motions act together to spin or rotate the expanding bubble in a clockwise fashion (clockwise as seen from the front).

Figure 28
Rotating the
Bubble

(From the Front)

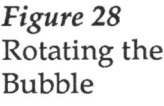
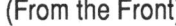
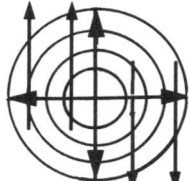

Vertical Flows

Resulting Rotation

This rotation or spinning is much like a slow speed centrifuge. Spinning of any medium causes the medium to hollow out in the center, forming a vortex. (This is what happens to the liquid in a food blender or to the water going down the bathtub drain.) The direction of the vortex is controlled by the direction of the upward and downward movement in the peripheral flows and the frontward motion is controlled by the helixes around the peripheral flows.

Figure 29
Forming the Vortices

The flow on the right moves upward and so does the right hand edge of the vortex. The left hand edge of the vortex moves down along with the vertical flow.   Thus the vertical flows mesh together with the vortices without clashing.

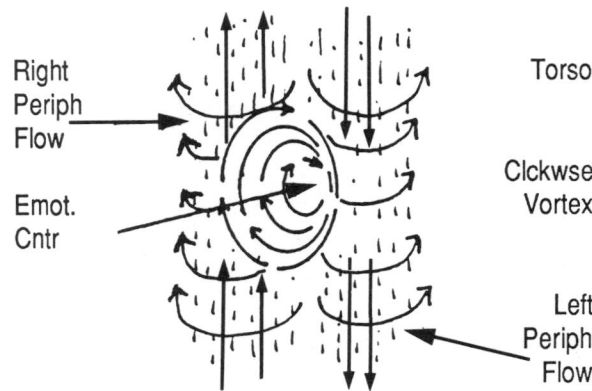

Right
Periph
Flow

Emot.
Cntr

Torso

Clckwse
Vortex

Left
Periph
Flow

COMPRESSION OF THE CENTERS.

Now, a problem occurs because the emotion
centers are so close together in the body.
The emotion from the centers is not free to
expand evenly in all directions. The result
is a compression of the field coming from
the centers into elongated, nearly elliptical
regions of emotion.

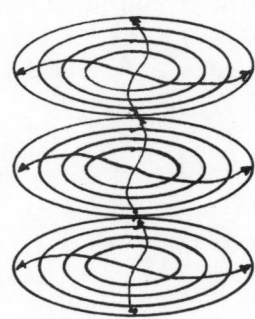

Figure 30 Compressed Centers

The principle movement of the field in the emotion centers is outward. However, the
rules that govern circulating fields demand that the frontward flow eventually return to
the starting point at its beginning (the spine). The portion of the physioemotional field
radiating out from the emotion center returns to its source, much like the water from a
recirculating fountain does. (Remember, this energy system is not like the sun, it is a
closed system, all parts of it flow in endless patterns.)

Figure 31 Return Flows

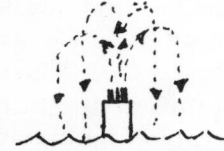

Circulating
Water
Fountain

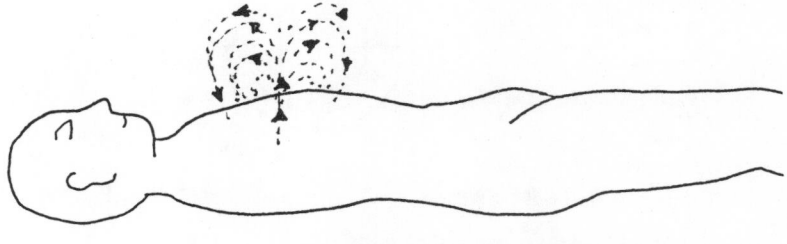

Circulating Energy at Emotion Center

Now, the compression effect mentioned earlier causes a problem with the return flows.
There is no problem for the part of the flow coming out of the sides of the center as there
is nothing to restrict the return, it follows the helix around the peripheral flows.

However, there is a problem for the portion
that would normally return at the top and
the bottom edges of the compressed center.
The return flows from adjacent centers try
to return at the same place and bump into
each other, overlapping in the process.

This results in **Bands of Emotion** that are
joined/separated by areas of interference, or
Blocking Centers which block the adjacent
emotions.

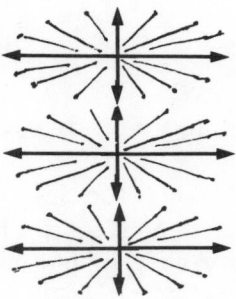

Figure 32 Blocking Segments
(Interferences Between Centers)

EMOTION REGIONS AND BLOCKING SEGMENTS

The results of elongation of the emotion centers into bands, or *emotion regions*, is shown here.

In the emotion regions, shown as the white areas, movement in the field is toward the front of the body, in the *blocking segments*, shown as the shaded areas, movement is toward the back.

Figure 33 Emotion Regions

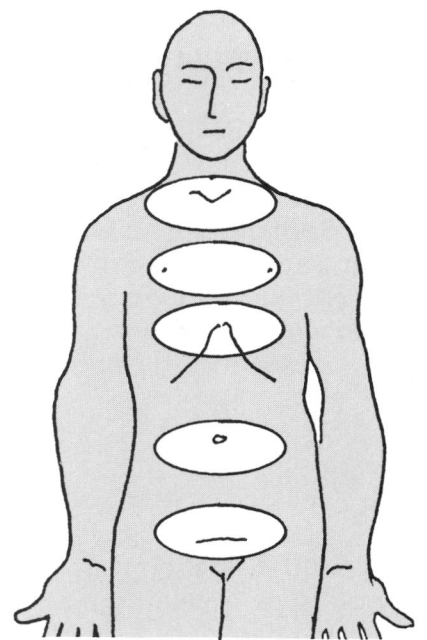

These overlapping areas produce the local skin color and body temperature shifts in response to emotional tension, or contraction, that are called **Reichian Bands** [30]*. The Reichian effect is the result of one emotion region being relaxed (with good capillary perfusion) and the adjacent area being constricted (with poor capillary perfusion).*

This overlapping and mixing of the return flows from the emotion centers is the *physiological* reason why we sometimes find ourselves in the position of loving someone so much we can't be angry at them while at the same time being so angry at them that we can't love them. The physiological repression of either love or anger represses the other. (This is why it is so difficult for the person who tries to be "in their heart" by repressing anger, to actually be in their heart. The anger is suppressed, but the suppressing action also affects the heart.) The same emotional lockup can occur between anger/fear and confidence/guilt and between confidence/guilt and sexual feeling.

This completes the theory you need to complete the Training. You may turn ahead to page 87 if you wish, and go on where you left off studying.

---

[30] Bands of pink and white observed in the torsos of some people when under emotional stress. Identified by Wilhelm Reich and noted by many practitioners of hands-on emotional release work.

POSTULATING ANSWERS TO SOME DIFFICULT QUESTIONS

(You may have wondered about some of these questions, however it is not at all necessary to know the answers in order to understand how SHEN works.)

WHAT HAPPENS WHERE THE ARM AND BODY FLOWS CROSS? When two flows come together, as happens when the arm flow crosses the peripheral flows, something has to give. *Even though we can't see the crossing of these flows because they are inside the body, we can deduce what they do because we know what magnetic fields do when they cross. Two magnetic fields crossing at right angles deflect in one of two patterns, depending upon polarity.*

Figure 34
Crossing Fields

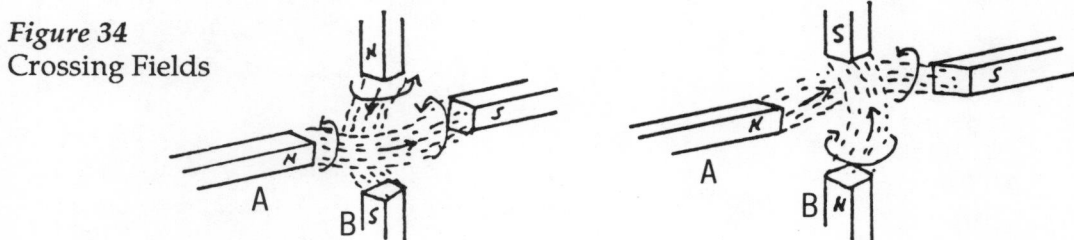

Notice that the rotary flow of "A" is going in the same direction as the main flow of "B" while the rotary flow of "B" is going in the same direction as the flow of "A". If either helix rotated in opposition to the other's main flow it would cause friction and neither flow could move freely. Because they interface this way, they create a synergistic action where, as one flow increases, its increased rotary action causes the other main flow to increase also. *This can easily be demonstrated. When a person brings their hands close together an increase in the field can be detected around their legs.*

Figure 35
Mixing
the Flows

normal
flow

Vertical
flow
increases

and

its helix
increases

Which

causes
the
horizontal
flow to
increase

Figure 36
The Combined Flows

When combined, the two vertical peripheral flows and the arm flow look like this: (Notice that all rotary flows coincide with the main flows in adjacent paths.)

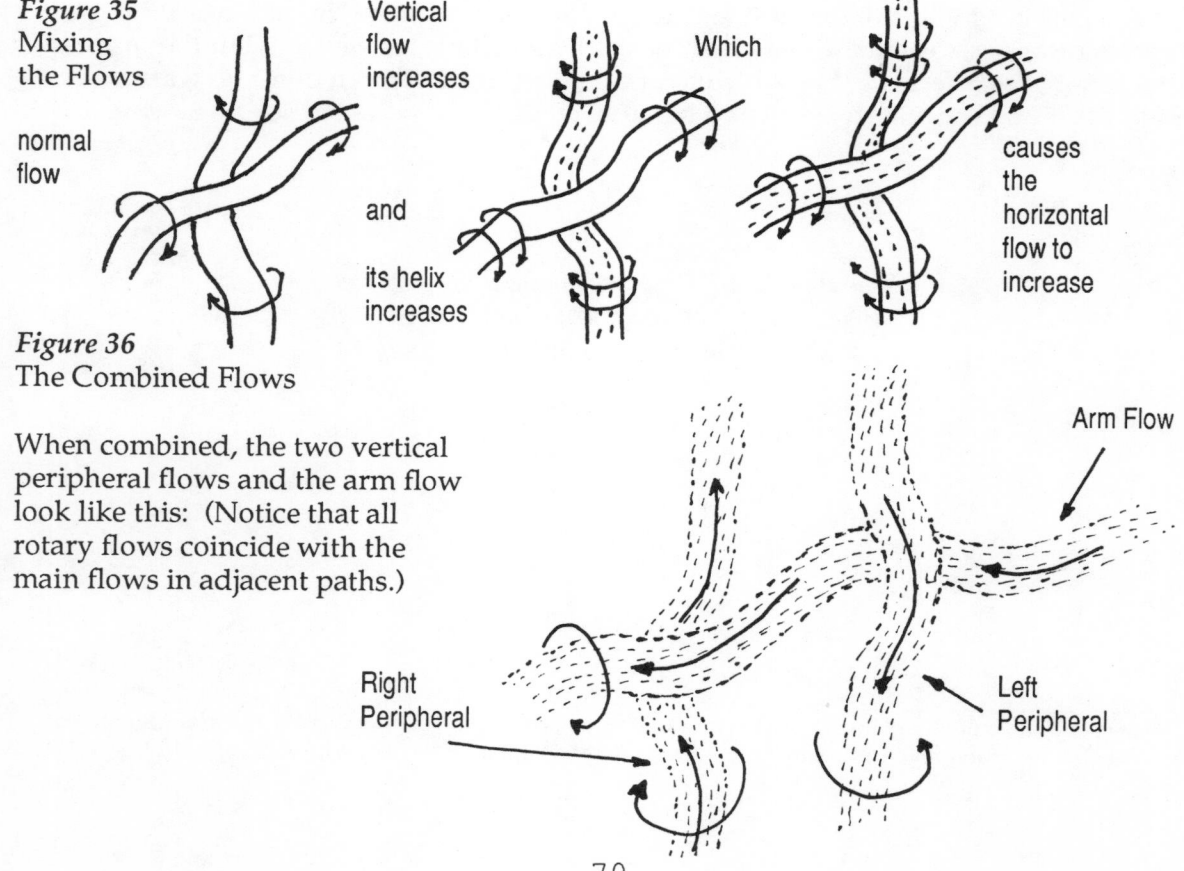

Arm Flow

Right
Peripheral

Left
Peripheral

WHAT DRIVES THE FIELD?

Something has to drive the field through the body. This crossing of flows is located at the lungs and lung action and seems to cause a pumping action that activates the field. This is why the field effect at the hands increases as the breath rate increases. There is an action that occurs in electrical transformers and coils that can explain this.

When a current begins to flow through an electrical conductor, or wire, in a transformer coil, it produces an expanding electrical field around the wire. When the current is stopped the field collapses and in collapsing, *causes a new voltage and current to be produced in the wire and in wires next to it.*

Figure 37
Transformer Action

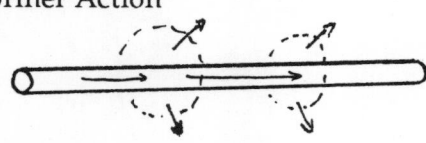 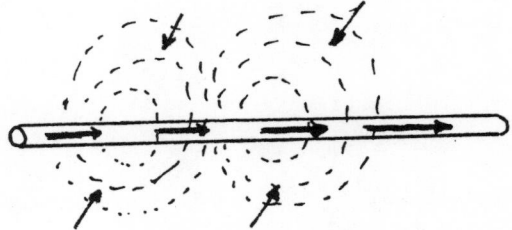

Increasing current produces an expanding field   Collapsing field induces a new current

A similar action by the lungs produces the flow (current or movement) in the physioemotional field in the body. When the lungs expand to take in a breath the field expands also because the field moves as the body moves. When it does, the field is driven in its normal pattern. *It is the expansion and contraction of the peripheral flows and the arm flow that drives the field.*

The expansion and contraction occur each time the chest and abdomen expand and contract during breathing. Each breath not only brings air into the lungs but also moves the field through the entire physical body, providing *life* and the possibility of emotion.

Figure 38
Breath
and the
"Pump"

field
expands

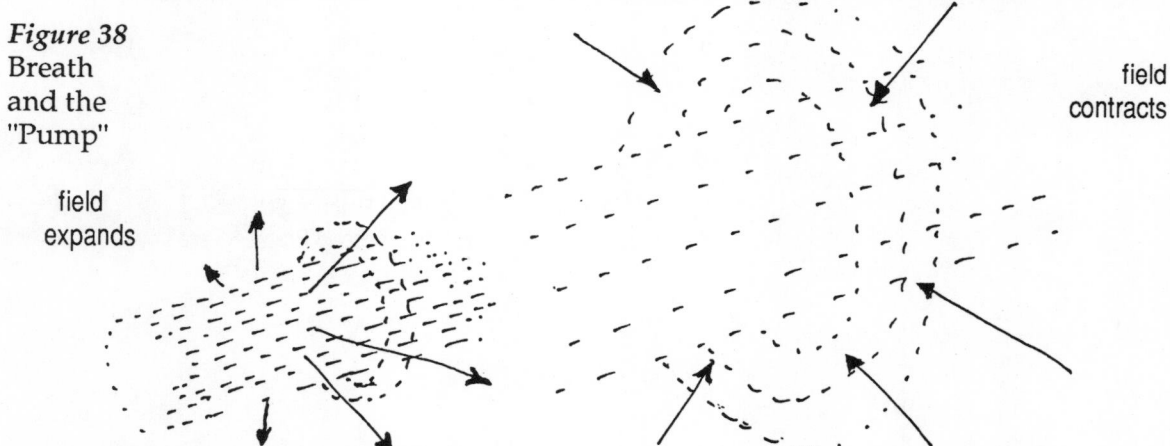

field
contracts

The contraction/expansion action causes the field to flow at right angles through the body. That is, as the chest moves in or out, the flow moves vertically through the body, or across the arms.

REVIEW OF

CHAPTER 8

1. Draw the pattern of the flows in this figure.

2. And indicate the five emotion centers.

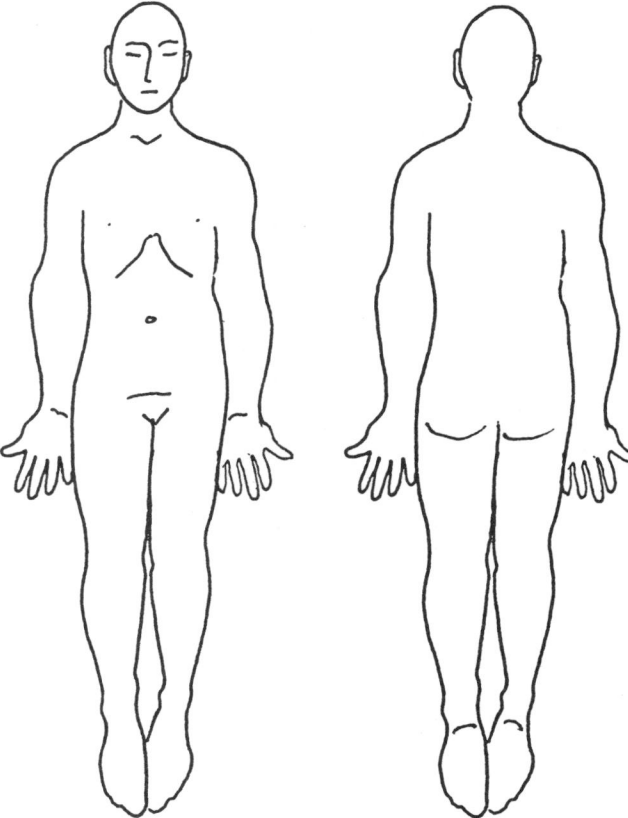

3. The field moves:
   a. With the nerves.
   b. With the meridians.
   c. Through all body tissue.
   d. Counter to blood flow.

4. Emotion Radiates:
   a. To the sides.
   b. To the front.
   c. All around the body.
   d. In definite patterns.

5. The mechanism that pumps the field to keep it going is:
   a. The action of the lungs.
   b. Rotary hand motions.
   c. A deep mental process.
   d. Leg motion.

SECTION III
LEARNING TO DO SHEN
Page 73

*There is much more to SHEN than simply placing your hands on a
person, and much more than just placing them in haphazard or random
positions around an emotion region or trauma site. If it were all that
simple, this section wouldn't be needed, but if it were all that
complicated, the section couldn't have been written.*

CHAPTER 9   **BASIC SHEN** _____ 75
Learning to Sense the Field, 75. Determining the Direction of your Arm/Hand Flow, 76. General Instructions
for Doing SHEN Flows, 78. First Practice Session (Day 1), 80. Second Practice Session (Day 1), 82.

Review Questions for Chapter 9, 84.

First Outside Practice Session, 85.
Second Outside Practice Session, 86.

CHAPTER 10   **SHEN FLOWS AT THE EMOTION CENTERS** _____ 87
Definitions, 87. Working With the Emotion Regions, 88. Shoulder/Head Flows, 90. First Practice Session
(Day 2), 91. Notations, 92. Second Practice Session (Day 2), 93. Transverse Flows, 93. Crown Flows,
94. Third Practice Session (Day 2), 94.

Third Outside Practice Session (Solar Plexus) 95.
Fourth Outside Practice Session (Heart) 96.
Fifth Outside Practice Session (Pubic) 97.
Sixth Outside Practice Session (Throat and Root) 98.

CHAPTER 11   **ADVANCED SHEN PROCEDURES** _____ 99
Expanded Root and Crown Flows, 99. Frontal Flows, 100. First Practice Session (Day 3), 101. Flows at
the Sides, 102. Combining Flows Through Two Centers, 103. Second Practice Session (Day 3), 105.
Points to Remember, 105.

Review of Chapter 10 and 11, 106.

This section comprises the main text for the SHEN Training Seminars. The course comprises three training days which are usually scheduled with two weeks between Day 1 and Day 2 and four weeks between Day 2 and Day 3.

Six outside practice sessions are assigned, one during each of the six intervening weeks, in addition to the practice during class. If you wish to accelerate, you can do as many as three outside practice sessions in a week. More than that will likely result in confusion.

If you study this on your own you will need a partner or partners to practice with as the training is based on each student receiving as well as giving all the practice SHEN sessions outlined in the course. Since SHEN work does release emotions in a unique way, it is important to have experienced the process fully in order to properly assist your patient/client through these releases. If you yourself have not had the unique experience of SHEN, you will likely falter at exactly the times that will fail your client.

By following the lessons in this section, you will be guided through the process in easy to assimilate steps so that you can absorb the entire experience quickly and be completely comfortable with the process.

CHAPTER 9

BASIC SHEN
(Training for Day One and the
First Two Outside Practice Sessions.)

LEARNING TO SENSE THE FIELD

Before learning to do flows through another person you will first need to learn how to detect or "feel" the field with your hands.

Step 1. To start, place your hands, palms open and facing, about eighteen inches apart. (Your partner(s) should be doing the same thing with their hands.) Slowly bring your hands together and see if you feel "something" between them.

Figure 39 Sensing the Field

Now, this will be a subtle sensation and you may miss it at first if you are not careful. It will most likely feel like a subtle pressure or change in heat. Some report that it feels like tingles, electricity, pressure or magnetism. It is not at all important that you perceive it the same way as someone else does.

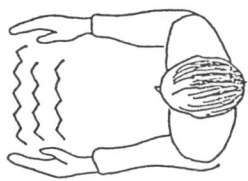

In fact, it is not even vital that you sense it at all. *A good friend of mine who has been doing SHEN for a number of years rarely, if ever, senses the field with his hands and it has not prevented him from doing very good work.* However, being sensitive to the energy does help.

Step 2. Do this exercise again and stop at the point where you sense the "something". Now begin to rotate your hands in small circles (about ten inches) with the palms facing and notice if and how the sense of the field changes. Does it increase? Or decrease? Then:

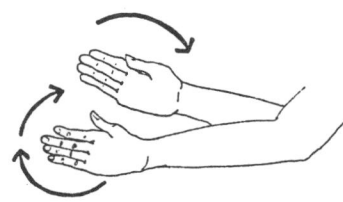

Figure 40 Rotating the Hands

Step 3. Bring your hands apart, perhaps two feet, and slowly bring them together again, noticing where they are when you begin to feel the sensation you felt previously. Is the distance the same? Or farther apart? Closer together? Most people find that the sensations and the distance between the hands has increased, often quite noticeably.

Rotating your hands in this fashion energizes and increases the field between them. *The process is much like stroking an iron nail across the face of a magnet. As you do, the nail becomes magnetized and becomes able to pick up small bits of iron.* Some SHEN practitioners do this process for a few minutes just before starting a SHEN session.

Do not worry about how strong the sensations are at this time, they will increase markedly during the training. Also, you are not likely to have the same type or amount that your partner, or anyone else, gets so you will not be able to judge your experience by theirs.

Over time you will find that the sensations will become very good indicators of the strength of the flows you are sending through the person you are working with. You may also find that there are differences in the quality of the sensations you perceive when your hands are over physical pain, over emotional pain or over physical tension in the body. What is important, now, is that you begin to catalogue the types of sensations that you yourself receive and relate them to what they mean.

DETERMINING THE DIRECTION OF YOUR ARM/HAND FLOW

As was mentioned in an earlier chapter, most people have arm/hand flows that move out of the palm of the right hand and back into the left. Of all those who have trained in SHEN, about one percent have flows going the other way, out the left and into the right. We do not have an explanation for the difference at this time, but do know that it has nothing to do with being physically right or left-handed. It is absolutely necessary to know the direction of your flows or you may end up doing everything backwards. To determine your flow direction:

Step 1. Face your partner and do the rotary hand exercise that you just did in Step 2 (Figure 40). Then place your hands up and facing out with about eight inches between your hands. (Caution: Do not try this where there is a draft.)

Step 2. Your partner places the palm of his or her right hand about three inches in front of your right palm.

Figure 41 Determining Arm Flow Direction

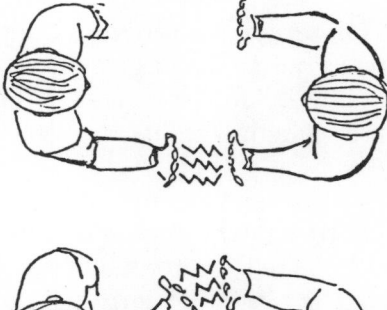

Step 3. Without moving your hands, will the energy to flow out of your right hand into their palm. (Willing is the mental effort that occurs just before your body reacts physically.) Have your partner notice how that feels.

Step 4. Then, your partner moves their right hand over to about three inches in front of your left hand.

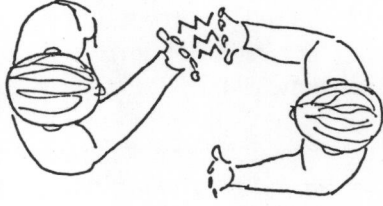

Step 5. Now will the energy to flow out of your left hand. Have your partner compare what they feel with what they felt at your right hand.

Step 6. When you have finished, have your partner tell you which was stronger. The stronger flow is your natural flow and the direction that you will always use.

If the difference between your flows was too weak to tell, or if your partner has difficulty sensing them, try this same process while having your partner sense the flow strength with his or her *left* palm.

If your partner still can't tell for sure, assume that you are a right handed sender (remember almost everybody is) and have your hands re-checked after you have done several practice sessions. *Incidently, every left-handed sender that I know has had extremely strong flows from the very beginning, there has never been any question about their direction.*

After you have been checked it is time to check your partner's hands.

CAUTION: This is **the only time** you should attempt to "effort" or "will" the energy to flow from your hand(s). Doing this during a SHEN session will tire you quickly and you will find that, contrary to what you might expect, your flows will not be as strong as they will be when you just let them flow naturally. You should not try to "visualize" the flows moving through the patient/client's body, either, for the same reason.

IS IT SUGGESTION - OR IS IT REAL?
This is a good time to determine if you are imagining the effect just because you see your partner's hand in front of yours. You and your partner will need a sheet of newspaper to do this.

Step 1. Drape a piece of newspaper over the edge of a table.

Step 2. Both you and your partner energize your hands.

Step 3. Sit in a chair close to the paper and hold your hand still, about two inches behind the paper, palm open and facing the paper.

Step 4. Your partner places his or her sending hand about two inches from the paper in front of your palm. (The paper is in between.)

Step 5. Your partner moves their palm up, down and across your palm and fingers, *stopping in between movements.*

Notice what you feel. Report changes in sensation to your partner for confirmation.

Step 6. Your partner can point his or her finger tips at your palm and move the tips across your palm, stopping between movements, if you wish.

Figure 42
Suggestion or Real?

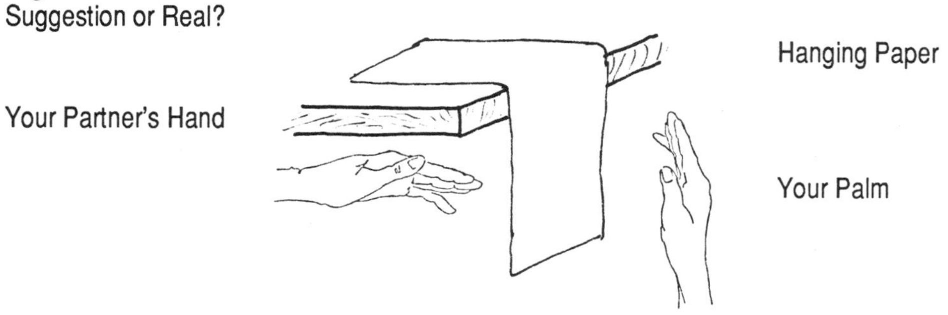

Your Partner's Hand

Hanging Paper

Your Palm

GENERAL INSTRUCTIONS FOR DOING SHEN FLOWS

A.   The flows do not proceed instantly from your sending hand through the patient/client and into your receiving hand. It may take up to several minutes for this to occur. The time involved depends on the distance between your hands, the physioemotional tension in the person's body and the strength of your flows.

In the future, when you have become sensitive to the sensation of the flow entering your hand, you will know when it is time to move to the next part of the procedure. However, for now, plan to keep your hands at each of the segments for about three minutes.

B.   Remember that while relaxation of specific body regions is a major part of SHEN work, the state of the person's whole body tension (or relaxation) will contribute to this regional relaxation. Anything that can be done to make the patient/client comfortable will help with the process.

If supine, place a rolled towel under their knees; use a thin pillow beneath their head if wish. If prone, wedge the towel under the front of their ankles. You may need to elevate their abdomen if they have low back pain.

Use relaxing music and dim the lights. However, do not use the person's, or your own favorite music. Often a person's favorite music is stimulating rather than relaxing. Quiet ocean tapes, *white noise* and other non-evocative music are all useful in blanking out whatever noise is in the background and in helping the patient/client relax.

C.   If you won't be able to move freely around the patient/client because they are on a couch or narrow bed that is against a wall or other obstruction, be sure that their head is to your left so that you can do the flow up their spine correctly. (If you are a left handed sender their head needs to be on your right.)

D.   Pay attention to your breathing. If your stomach or chest get tight or if your breathing gets shallow, begin to breathe regularly and fully, filling your lower stomach. (Your breath rate often stops or slows when you get tense about what to do next, or when the patient/client releases emotion). Remember, movement of the energy through your body is dependent upon the pumping that occurs when you breathe.

Figure 43
Hot Spot

E.   The most active part of the hand is not the fingers but a silver dollar size area in the palm.

When doing flows, be sure the palm is centered where you want the greatest effect.

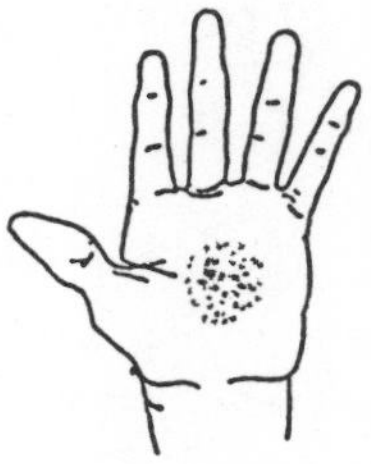

F.   Imagine that there is an arrow between your hands with the arrow head in the palm of your **Receiving** (Left) hand and the feathers in the palm of your **Sending** (Right) hand. If you match this imaginary arrow with the flows in the person's body, you will always be correct.

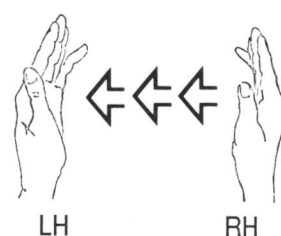

Figure 44 Direction of Flow

LH   RH

G.   Keep an easy posture. You may sit, kneel or stand depending upon the height of the bed you are using. Get centered comfortably. When your body gets stiff you can rock back or forward into a slightly different position, to ease the strain. Remember not to put any pressure on the person when you do this - and don't rock back and forth continually.

Do not twist your spine in order to reach to a new segment, instead get up, move to a new position, re-center and relax. (If you are twisted when the person releases emotion, you will catch it right in your back.) And, keep your wrists relaxed, do not lean your weight on the person.

H.   Do **not** leave your hands on the person when shifting the rest of your body to a new position. (SHEN is not like massage, keeping one hand in place during SHEN will jostle the person and break the deep state that they may be in.)

Figure 45 Merging Flows

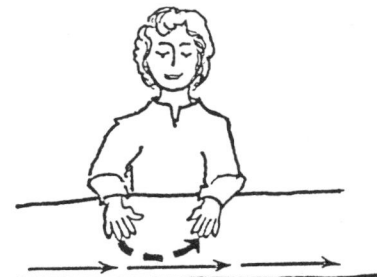

I.   This shows how the flow leaves your sending hand and enters the person's body, moves through it in conjunction with their own flow and returns to your receiving hand. *NOTICE THAT THEIR FLOWS DO NOT MOVE THROUGH YOUR BODY.*

J.   Try not to talk with the person you are working with during the session. Remember that you are disturbing the person and ruining the relaxation effect. (Sometimes the patient/client will practically insist on dialoguing because they are a bit afraid. If they do, tell them that it breaks your concentration.)

Figure 46 Shorting the Arms

K.   If it is necessary to cross your arms to reach the segments on the other side of their body to get the direction of the flow correct, do not let your arms touch or you will short out the circuit and the flow won't get to your hands.

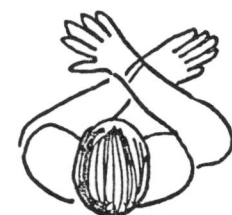

NOTE: *The instructions for the practice sessions that follow assume that your **Right Hand** is your **Sending Hand** and your **Left Hand** is your **Receiving Hand**. Those who are left handed senders will have to convert.*

FIRST PRACTICE SESSION (DAY 1)   PERIPHERAL & ARM FLOWS
(Allow an hour and a half if you and your partner both practice.)

NOTE: *Lay this chart on the person's torso, oriented to their head, use it as a "road map".*

Figure 47
PERIPHERAL & ARM FLOWS
(Supine Position)

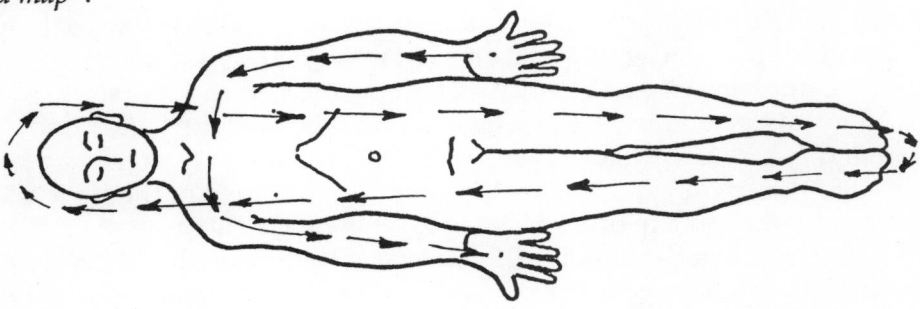

(You won't do the arm flows in this Session)

Remember match arrow between your hands (Fig. 44) with the arrows on his/her body.

Read through the instructions on this and the next page before you start

1.   Begin at any point but bottom of right foot is a good place to start.
2.   Your hands should be under, or at the sides of, the body, not on top.
3.   Do segments of reasonable length:
     a. Foot (RH) to knee (LH)
     b. Knee (RH) to Hip (LH)
     c. Hip (RH) to shoulder (LH)

It is important not to leave gaps. Here is how to prevent that:

Figure 48 Overlapping the Segments

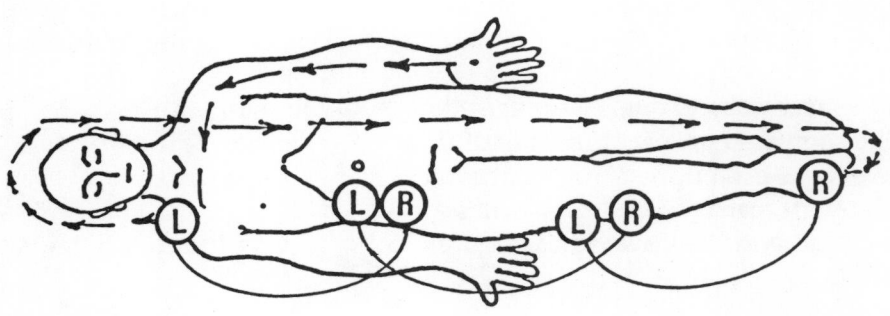

80

d. The loop around the head

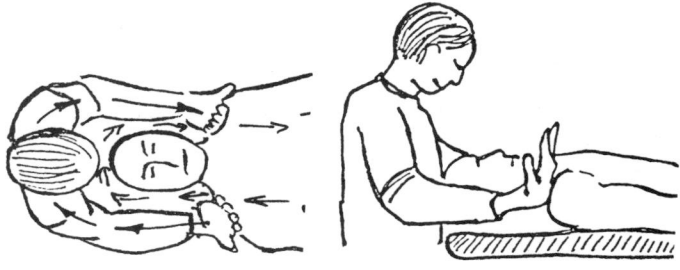

Figure 49 Head Loop

This is one time when it is easy to confuse
yourself as to where your palms should face
when doing a flow. In order for your flows
to match the flow around the head, the
backs of your hands must rest on the
shoulders, as shown here. Then go on:

  e. Shoulder (RH) to hip (LH)

  f. Hip (RH) to knee (LH)

  g. Knee (RH) to foot (LH)

4.   Finish the session by leaving the palm of your Left Hand on the bottom of the
person's left foot, and place your Right Hand on the bottom of the right foot, so as to do
a flow through the entire body.

5.   Hold your hands in each segment for about three minutes.

6.   It is not likely that emotion will surface during this session but it might. If it does let
it complete its course, it will pass quickly.

7.   Remember, pay attention to your breath - keep it deep and full.

   Now, go back to step one, energize your hands, and begin the session.

When you have completed the session, give your partner some time to come back to
normal and sit up.

NOTE: If your partner feels lightheaded after receiving the session, have them sit
upright in a chair, with their back straight and breathe deeply into the lower stomach,
filling the navel area for a minute or so. If YOU feel lightheaded after giving a session, it
is probably because you were nervous and fell into shallow breathing. A few good deep
breaths should overcome that. (I have had students who became nervous because they
were a little frightened about the possibility of some of their own emotion surfacing.
Once they experienced that the release of emotion through SHEN is very different from
keeping it pent up and then pouring it out on the world, their nervousness disappeared.)

Now it is your partner's turn to give you this session. After your partner has given you
your session the two of you can compare observations. You might notice:

A.   If the sensations you felt were the same in all parts of your body.
B.   Were your hand sensations the same at all segments of their body.
C.   How did these impressions coordinate with your partner's.

   Now you are ready to go on to the Second Practice Session

SECOND PRACTICE SESSION (DAY 1)   ARM & SPINE FLOWS
(Allow an hour if you both practice this set.)

In this session you will do two sets of flows, Arm Flows and Spine Flows

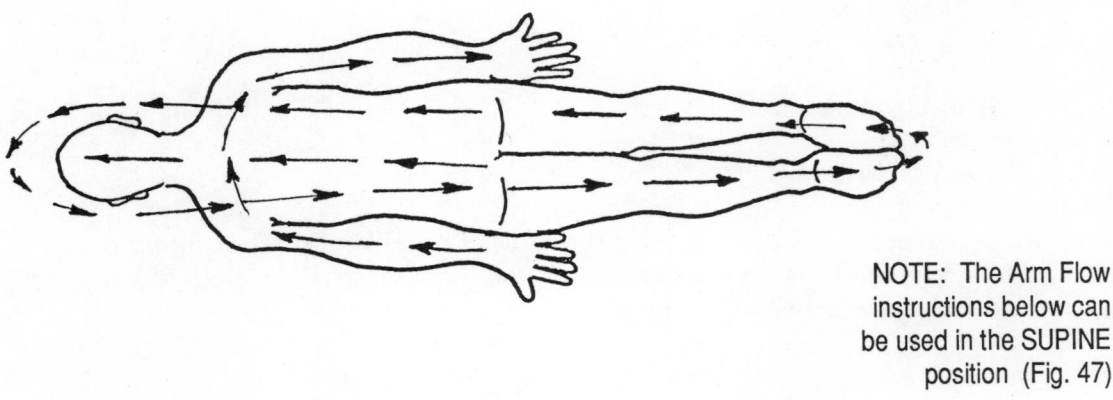

Figure 50
ARM, SPINE & PERIPHERALS
(Prone Position)

NOTE: The Arm Flow
instructions below can
be used in the SUPINE
position (Fig. 47)

SPINE FLOW: The spine flow begins at the caudal ganglia, just under the tail bone and flows on to the crown of the head.   To begin, you:

1.   Center the palm of your RH at the lower buttocks crease and center the palm of your LH on the spine, just above the buttocks, for three minutes. Then, leaving your RH where it is,
2.   Place your LH palm on the spine at middle of the back for 3 minutes,
3.   Then palm of LH on the spine at the rise of the shoulders, 3 minutes,
4.   Then palm of LH on the back of the neck for 3 minutes,
5.   Finally, place the LH on the top of **(not the back of)** the head for 3 Min.

   As soon as you finish with the SPINE FLOWS, continue with the ARM FLOWS

6.   Place your RH on their left hand and your LH on the top of his/her left shoulder for 3 minutes. Then:
7.   Place your RH on the outside of their left shoulder and your LH on the outside of his/her right shoulder for 3 minutes. Then:
8.   Place your RH on top of their right shoulder and place your LH in his/her right hand for 3 minutes. Then:
9.   Leave your LH in his/her right hand, and do a complete arm flow by placing your RH in his/her left hand, for 3 minutes.

When both of you have finished you will probably wish to compare notes.   (In this session you combined two separate flows. They do not have to be done together, either can be done with any of the other flows you learn)

THIRD PRACTICE SESSION (DAY 1) EMOTION CENTER FLOWS & ROOT FLOWS
(Allow an hour and a half if you both practice this set.)

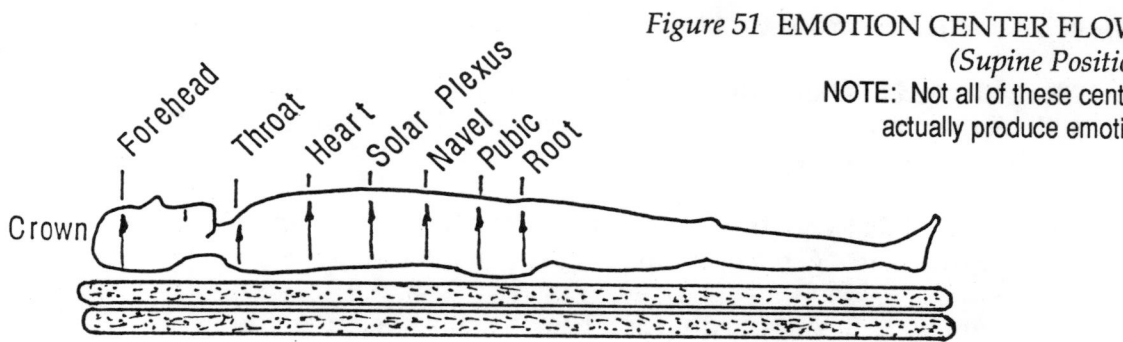

Figure 51 EMOTION CENTER FLOWS
(Supine Position)
NOTE: Not all of these centers
actually produce emotion.

You need double pads for these flows. Place your RH between the cushions and padded table, couch or bed. Otherwise your hand will cause the person discomfort. Also it will be squashed by the weight of the body. (You can take couch cushions and place them on a bed or massage table.)

Place your Right Hand behind the spine at the emotion center you wish to work with and your Left Hand on the front of the same center.

Do a:
1. Flow thru the Root (hand above pad for this one)   for 3 minutes
2. Flow thru Pubic Center (upper edge of pubic bone)   "
3. Flow thru Kath (just below navel)   "
4. Flow thru Solar Plexus (vee of the rib cage)   "
5. Flow thru Heart   "
6. Flow thru Throat (the notch) *careful, if touched there it feels like being choked*   "
7. Flow thru Forehead   "

Figure 52

ROOT FLOWS
(Supine Position)
These flows connect the Spine
Flow with the Emotion Centers

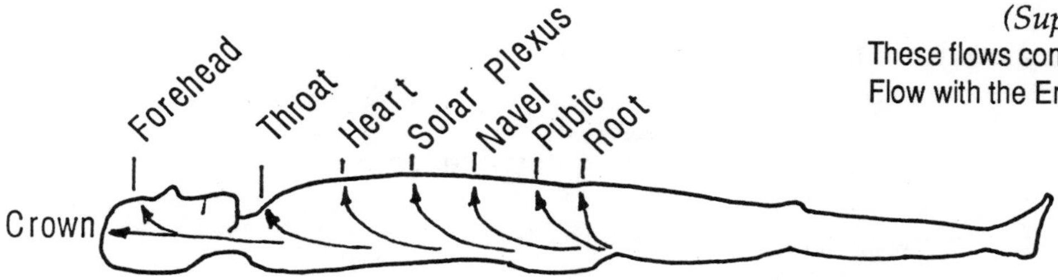

Then:
8. Place (and leave) Right Hand under buttocks, at the crease, palm up & Place LH above your RH, at Root (palm down on centerline) for 3 min
9. Then place LH on upper edge of pubic bone   "
10 Then place LH just below Navel (Kath)   "
11. Then place LH on vee at rib cage (Solar Plexus)   "
12. Then place LH on Heart   "
13. Then place LH at Throat, **but not touching**   "
14. Then place LH on Forehead   "
15. Then place LH on Crown   "

The SHEN flows used in therapy combine portions of the basic flows that you have just learned along with others you will learn in the future.

Now that you have learned the basic SHEN flows you need to practice them because:

1. You will need to know where the flows go in the body without having to look them up all the time. The advanced SHEN procedures are built on this fundamental knowledge.

2. You will find that your own flows will get much stronger, perhaps two to three times stronger, as you do the next two trade sessions.

3. Your own body field is freed up and begins to flow better as you receive the sessions. (This helps strengthen your arm flows, also.)

4. Your hands will become much more sensitive to the flows and you will begin to be able to sense when the flows begin to come through. This is quite helpful in doing effective therapeutic work with SHEN.

* * * * *

REVIEW OF
CHAPTER 9

1. What should you do if you feel light-headed during or after giving a SHEN session?

2. What happens when your breath rate slows down?

3. Where should you position the person's head before you start: To your Left or to your Right?

4. Where do your palms face when doing the head loop?

5. Why is it detrimental to "will" the energy to flow, or to visualize it flowing through the body, or out your sending hand?

FIRST OUTSIDE PRACTICE SESSION
(About two hours is needed for you and your partner to exchange)

1. Do the Peripheral Flows

Figure 53
ARM, SPINE & PERIPHERALS
(Prone Position)

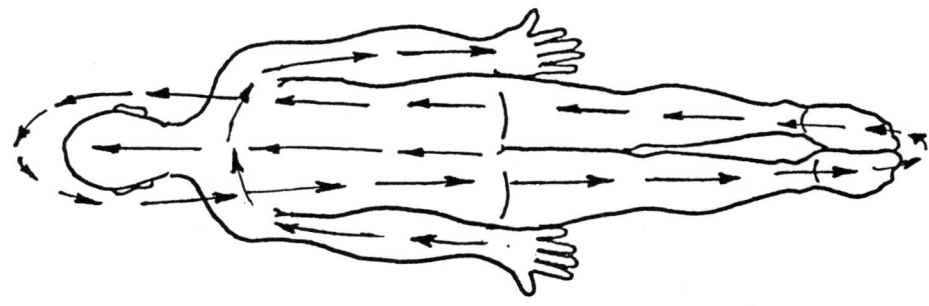

Figure 54 Head Loop

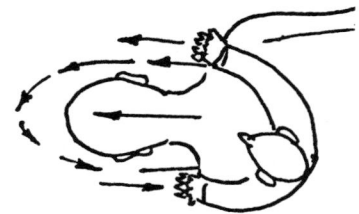

This picture shows you standing at the side, instead of in front as you did in Fig. 49, p. 81. (The flow is the same.)

2. And do the Arm Flows When finished, your partner turns over and

3. You end with the Root Flows

Figure 55 ROOT FLOWS
(Supine Position)

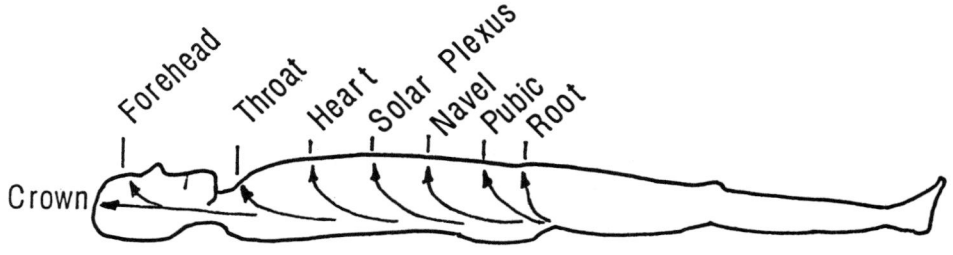

SECOND OUTSIDE PRACTICE SESSION
(You will need about two hours for you and your partner to exchange)

You will need double padding for this session. (Remember, you can take couch cushions and place them on a bed or massage table.)

1. Peripheral Flows

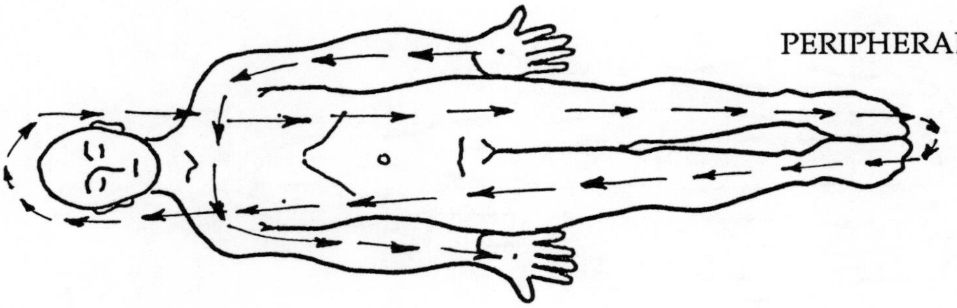

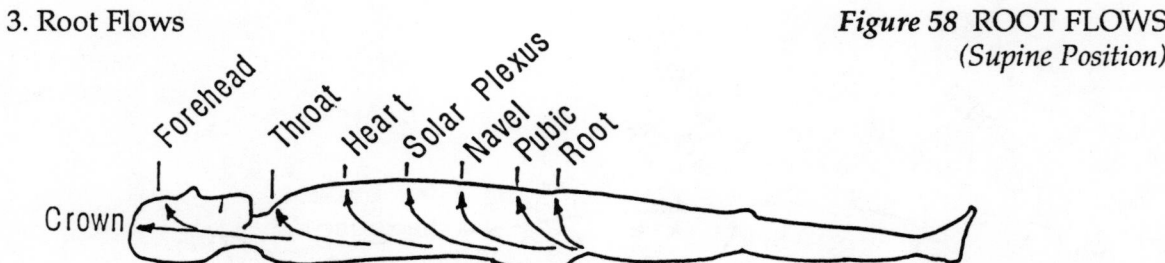

Figure 56
PERIPHERAL & ARM FLOWS
(Supine Position)

(Remember to do the Head Loop)

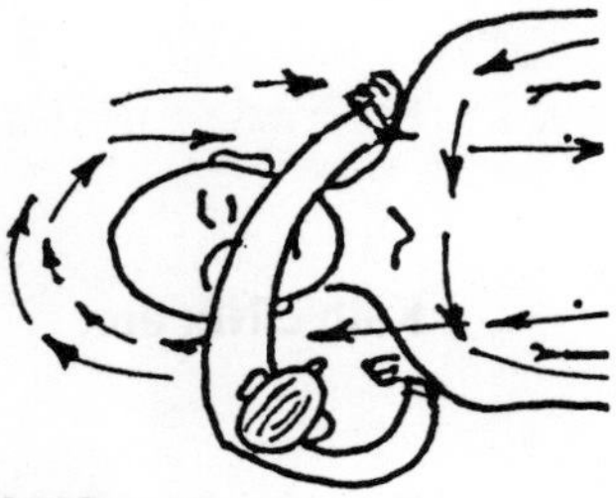

2. Emotion Center Flows
(Supine Position)

Figure 57 EMOTION CENTER FLOWS

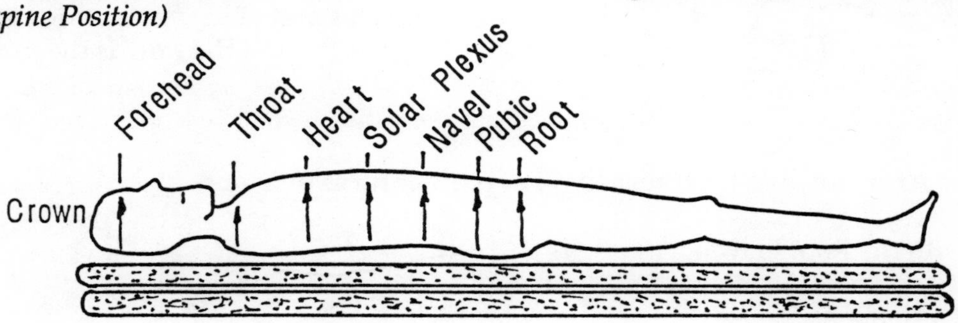

3. Root Flows

Figure 58 ROOT FLOWS
(Supine Position)

NOTE: *Practice on as many people as you can, your friends will love it.*

CHAPTER 10

SHEN FLOWS AT THE EMOTION REGIONS
(Training for Day Two and the
next four Outside Practice Sessions.)

Whether your interest in SHEN is for use in chronic pain, psychosomatic or behavioral medicine, in working with clients during emotional trauma, depression or for emotional growth with normal people, you will be working primarily with the emotion centers in very precise ways.

To do this effectively, you will need to be quick and efficient. The specific clinical procedures you will learn later on are all based on unique ways of releasing physioemotional tensions around the emotion centers, and combining these releases in an organized fashion that will be of best assistance to the patient/client.

At this time: Turn back to Chapter 8, Page 64 and read the indicated section. When you have finished, turn back to this page and continue.

Figure 59 Some Definitions

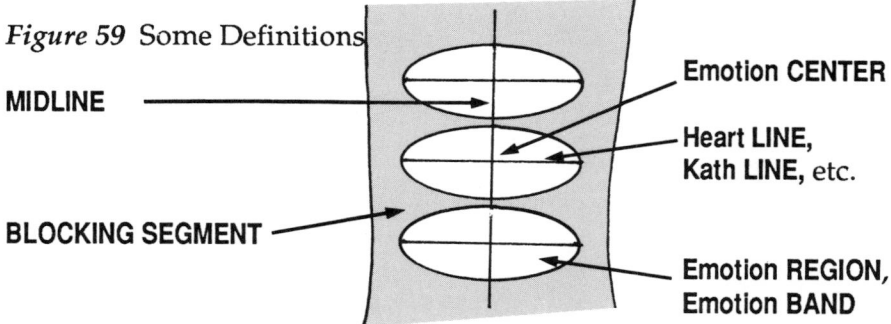

MIDLINE

BLOCKING SEGMENT

Emotion CENTER

**Heart LINE,
Kath LINE, etc.**

**Emotion REGION,
Emotion BAND**

It is extremely important that you know the exact center of the region you wish to work with. If you don't you will be trying to do flows in opposition to the body's normal flow and very little will happen.

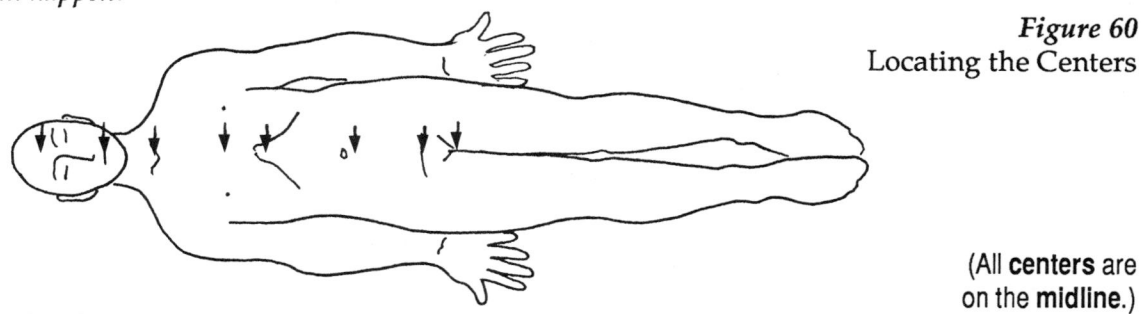

Figure 60
Locating the Centers

(All **centers** are
on the **midline**.)

Forehead	An inch above the eyebrows.
Mouth	Upper jaw line.
Throat	At the notch where the sternomastoids join the sternum.
Heart	Midway between the Throat Center and the xophoid process.
Solar Plexus	At the xiphoid process (the cartilage below the sternum).
Kath	An inch below the navel, on a line with the iliac crests.
Pubic	At the upper edge of the pubic bone.
Root	At the junction of the legs/lower buttocks crease.

SHEN Flows are almost always applied in the same direction as the normal body flow. This helps the body flow to regain normalcy. This means that we will do some flows with the RH on the front of the body and the LH on the rear and other flows with the RH on the rear of the body and the LH on the front.

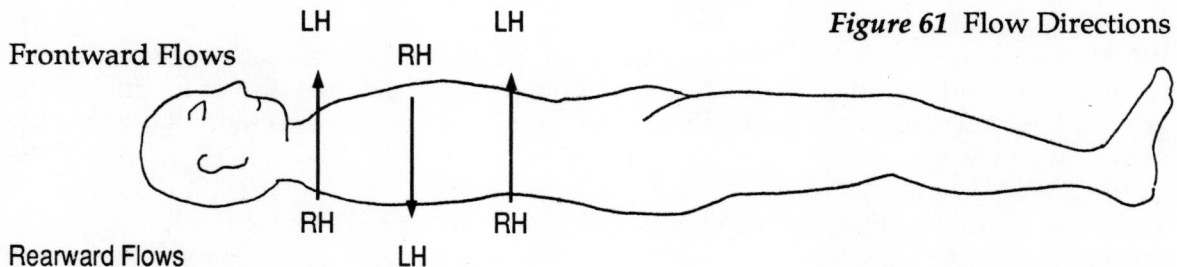

Figure 61 Flow Directions

WORKING EFFECTIVELY WITH THE ELONGATED REGIONS
You have probably guessed that merely doing a flow through the mid-point of these elongated emotion regions is not enough. To do a thorough job, at least three and, with larger people, possibly as many as five flows may be needed.

Figure 62
Multiple Flows

However, since moving the lower hand as is shown in figure 62 would be constantly disturbing to the person, we use a technique that is much less disturbing and is virtually as effective. In this method the lower hand is kept in the same position, at the spine, for all three flows. (These flows are usually called *Triples*.)

Figure 63 Simplified Triples

NOTE: When you do the triples, do not place your hands as far out to the sides as they are when you do Peripheral Flows.

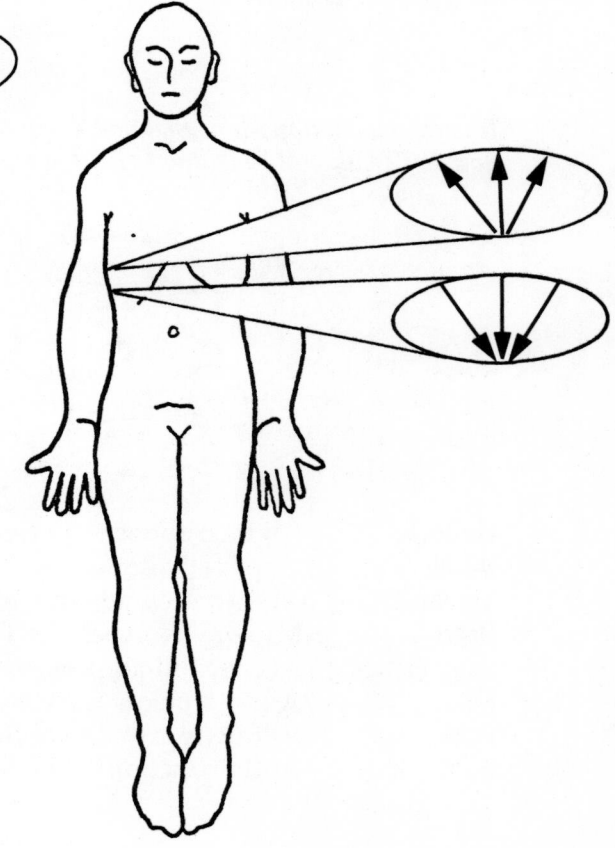

When doing Triples it is best to start with one on one side, then the one on the other side and last, the one in the center. (It is often easier to approach a tense area by first relaxing the edges, after they relax, relax the center.)

Figure 64 Locations of Frontward Triples
(At the Emotion Regions)

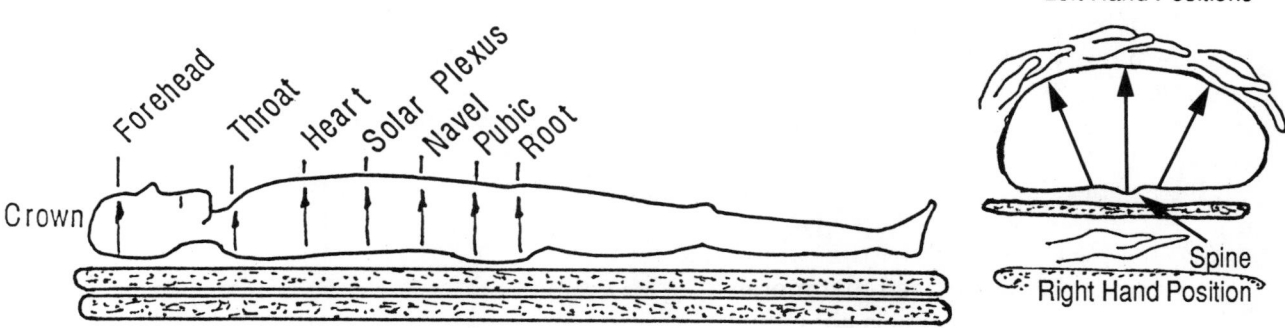

Figure 65 Locations of Rearward Triples
(At the Blocking Segments)

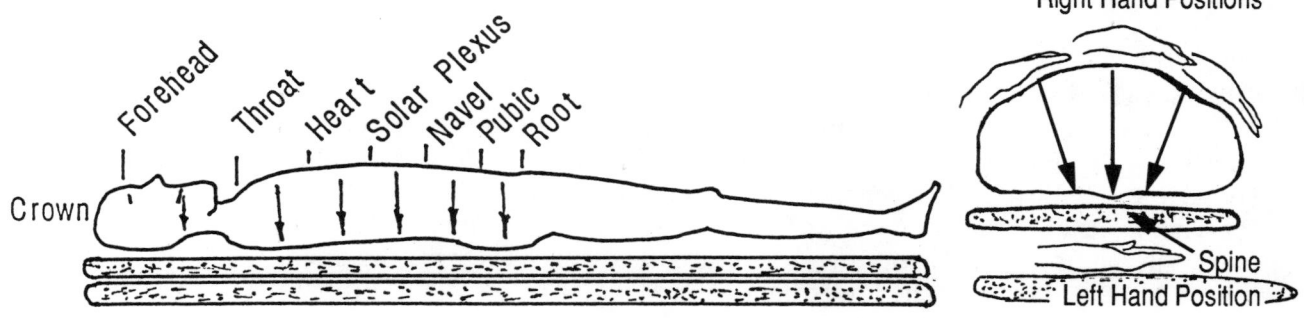

*(NOTE: Do **not** refer to the rearward flows as "reverse flows". **The flows are not reversed, as they are done in the normal direction for the segments.**)*

* * * * *

Most of the SHEN procedures you will use will be combinations of frontward and rearward flows. Usually, when working around an emotion center, you would do the rearward flows above and below first, and then follow with the frontward flows through the center.

The focus of the training so far has been on three things. Learning the basics, becoming aware of the sensations you feel with your hands and on the effects SHEN has on those you worked with. Building on that base, we can now begin finding ways to use those flows more effectively.

SHORTENING THE DAY 1 FLOWS.

The complete Peripheral Body Flows, Arm Flows and Root Flows are rarely used in their entirety in SHEN Therapy sessions. One reason is that too much time would be needed. It would take an hour to do all of these and then the real work would not have been started. However, parts of these flows are used quite effectively in almost every session.

You undoubtedly noticed that deep, general relaxation occurred during the sessions. Total body relaxation is a major factor in SHEN work. Without overall relaxation very little in the way of specific regional relaxation can occur. While there are times when it is possible to do SHEN procedures at the region of the deepest tension first and by relaxing those regions promote total body relaxation, there are many times when this does not work well. Sometimes the patient/client is apprehensive about SHEN, or is just frightened of relaxing. As a rule, it is best to go for general relaxation first and then follow with the specific regional work, especially during the patient/client's earlier SHEN sessions.

There are two specific body regions that contribute the most to overall tension. These are the shoulder girdle and the brain. (The brain is not always considered when thinking of physical tension but there is a direct correlation between Beta activity and tension. When Beta activity can be slowed the body relaxes rapidly. In any event, a simple procedure that combines parts of the Peripheral and Arm Flows is virtually as effective as the entire set, and the total time required is only nine or ten minutes. This leaves plenty of time for specific therapeutic work.

THE SHOULDER/HEAD FLOWS.

Step 1. This flow combines the first half of the Head Loop with a portion of the flow from the waist to the shoulder. Place your RH on the right side of the person's upper chest, in the hollow just under the clavicle (about half way between the Heart Line and the Throat Line). Then, place your LH with the palm facing to the right of the person and with the fingers pointing towards the head or down towards the table.

Figure 66 Shoulder/Head Flows

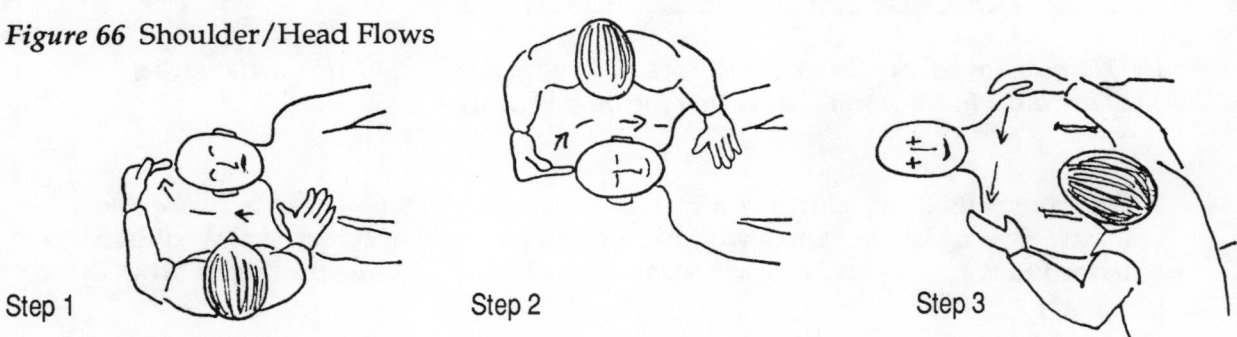

Step 1   Step 2   Step 3

Step 2. This is the mirror image of Step 1, with your RH at the top of the head and your LH on their left upper chest.

Step 3. Place your RH on the **outside** of their left shoulder and your LH on the **outside** of their right shoulder. (Not on top of the shoulders.)

Now you are ready to begin today's First Practice Session

FIRST PRACTICE SESSION (DAY 2) WORK AT THE KATH
(Allow about an hour and a half if you both practice this)

This session combines several flows, including the Shoulder/Head Flows and Triple Flows around the Kath. Most SHEN sessions include some work at the Kath. The Kath is the site of origin of emotions of confidence and accomplishment, emotions that are often submerged under repressed emotions of shame and guilt. Helping to uncover, release and complete the shame and guilt so that the desirable emotions of confidence and accomplishment can surface and be experienced is quite important. (Work at the Kath is central to the SHEN protocols for chronic low back pain, for irritable bowel syndrome and are part of the protocols for premenstrual and menstrual distress.)

In this session you do not have to maintain a strict three minute rule. If you feel a strong flow come through sooner than in three minutes, you can move on to the next segment - but try to be sure that the flow has really reached its maximum. Ideally, you should remain with the flow until it seems to taper off.

Figure 67 The KATH Session
First Part

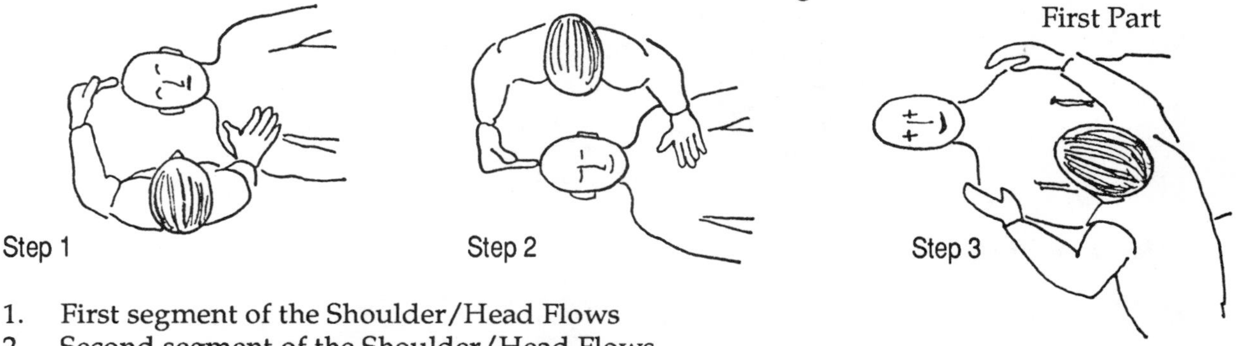

Step 1   Step 2   Step 3

1. First segment of the Shoulder/Head Flows
2. Second segment of the Shoulder/Head Flows
3. The shoulder segment of the Shoulder/Head Flows. Then:

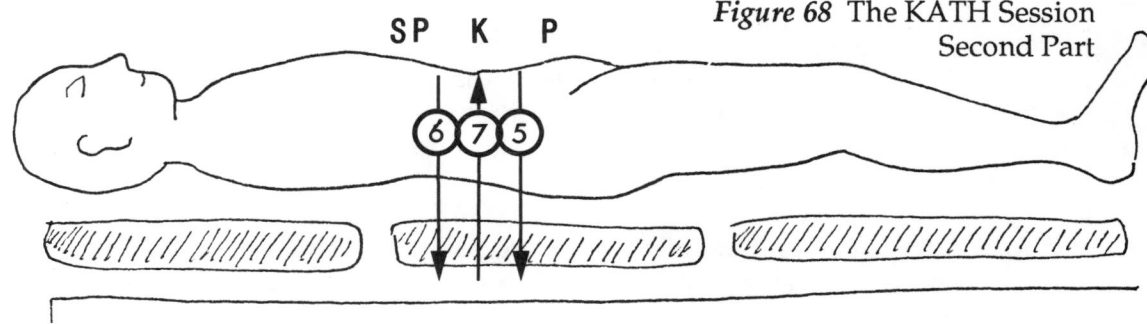

Figure 68 The KATH Session
Second Part

SP K P

⑥⑦⑤

4. Root to Kath
5. Rearward Triples, between the Pubic and Kath
6. Rearward Triples, between the Kath and Solar Plexus
7. Frontward Triples, at the Kath
8. Root to Kath   *(Steps 8 and 9 help to reintegrate*
9. Root to Crown   *the Regions with the main body flows)*
10. Feet (RH on right, LH on left)

When both sessions are finished, compare observations with your partner.

USING SHORTHAND NOTATIONS FOR SHEN FLOWS

By now you have become aware that when you are doing SHEN you often drift into a state where memory is not the sharpest and it is difficult to recall exactly when a significant release occurred after the session ends. Obviously, you cannot make copious notes at that time. This system of shorthand notations has been developed to help with that situation. *(This shorthand is used in the SHEN Protocols.)*

ANATOMICAL LOCATIONS

Crown	C	(Top of Head)
Forehead	F	(Just above the eyebrows)
Mouth	M	(Upper Jaw Line)
Throat	T	(Notch where the sternomastoids join the sternum)
	HT	(between Heart & Throat)
Heart	H	(Center of chest)
	SPH	(between Solar Plexus & Heart)
Solar Plexus	SP	(At the xophoid process - cartilage below sternum)
	KSP	(between Kath & Solar Plexus)
Kath	K	(Inch below navel, on line between the iliac crests)
	PK	(between Pubic & Kath)
Pubic	P	(Upper edge of pubic bone)
	RP	(between Root & Pubic)
Root	R	(Junction of legs/lower buttocks crease)

Figure 69 Precise Locations

Cross section of the
body at the Kath
viewed from the Feet

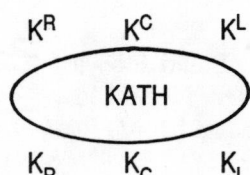

Except for the Forehead and Mouth, all emotion regions and blocking segments have three hand positions on the front and three on the back.
Use $^{\text{Superscript R,C or L}}$ for the upper hand positions and $_{\text{Subscript R,C or L}}$ for the lower hand positions. (Later you will use the lower positions.)

TRIPLE FLOWS

To record doing all three flows in a emotion region or blocking segment, follow the letter with a ^{Superscript} 3. For example: for three flows at the Heart use H^3, for three at the KSP Segment use KSP^3.

ROOT FLOWS

(The sequence of the letters indicates the direction of the flow. The location written first indicates the position of the the *sending* hand.)

(RH) (LH)

R-P	Root to Pubic	R-T	Root to Throat
R-K	Root to Kath	R-F	Root to Forehead
R-SP	Root to Solar Plexus	R-C	Root to Crown
R-H	Root to Heart		

LEARNING THE TRANSVERSE FLOWS

The Transverse Flows do not follow the movement of the physioemotional field through the body and are not used to directly restore normalcy to the field. These flows are performed at right angles to field movement and are used primarily to break physical tension in the body. They are often incorporated within specific SHEN Procedures and form a major part of SHEN work with chronic back pain.

The Transverse Flows are the easiest to learn. With one exception, place **either** hand on one side of the person's body and the other hand exactly opposite, on the other side of the body. *With most of these positions the flow direction doesn't matter, this is because they are across the field.* **The one where it does matter is through the shoulders - You should match your flow with the flow through the person's arms.**

SHORTHAND NOTATIONS FOR THE TRANSVERSE FLOWS

Examples: <R> <RP> <P> <PK> <K> <KSP> <SP> <SPH> <H> <HT> <T> <M>

SECOND PRACTICE SESSION (DAY 2) TRANSVERSE FLOWS
(This will take about an hour and a quarter if you both practice.)

(This one Transverse Flow is NOT Bi-Directional because it flows with the Arm Flow)

Figure 70 Transverse Flows
(Supine)
NOTE: Can be done prone as well

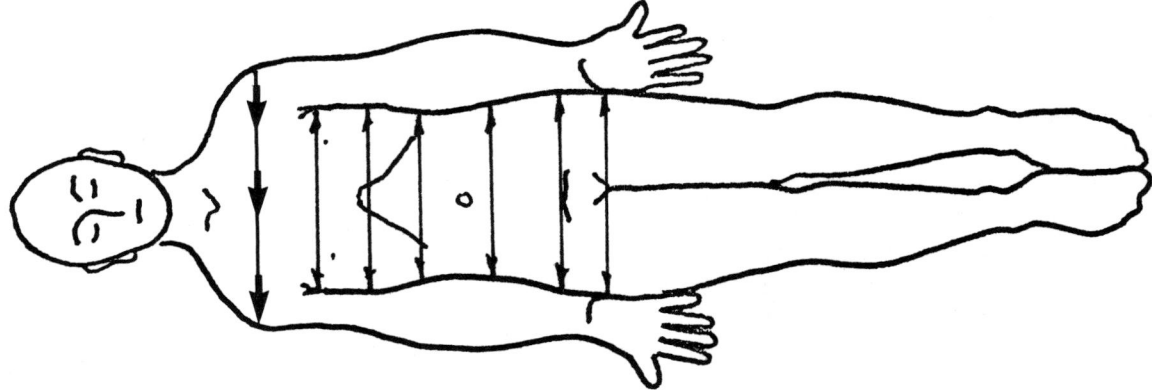

1. First segment of the Shoulder/Head Flows
2. Second segment of the Shoulder/Head Flows
3. The shoulder segment of the Shoulder/Head Flows. Then:
4. <R> (Across Root)
5. <P> (Across Pubic)
6. <K> (Across Kath)
7. <SP> (Across Solar Plexus)
8. <H> (Across Heart)
9. <T> (Across Throat)
10. <M> (Across Jaw line)
11. R-C (Root to Crown)

LEARNING THE CROWN FLOWS

To do the Crown Flows, place the LH (receiving hand) on the Crown and remains there while the RH (sending hand) is placed **between** any two emotion centers.   In a way, these are similar to the Root Flows.)

SHORTHAND NOTATIONS FOR THE CROWN FLOWS

As in the other Flows, the sending hand is always written at the left of the notation. In RP-C for example, the Right Hand is at RP, the Left Hand at the Crown.

THIRD PRACTICE SESSION (DAY 2) CROWN FLOWS
(Allow about three quarters of an hour for you both to practice)

Figure 71 Crown Flows   Right Hand Positions

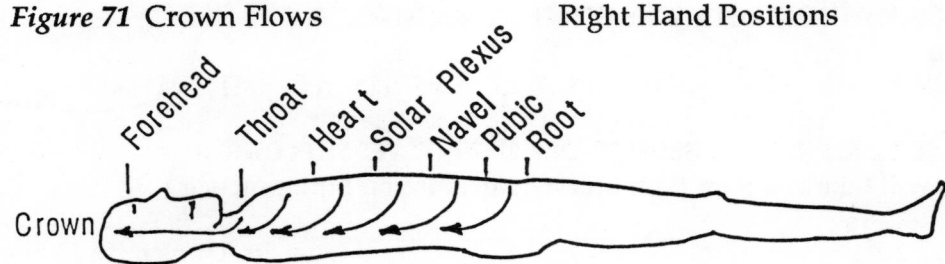

Your LH remains on Crown, place the RH successively at M, HT, SPH, KSP, PK, RP.

(RH) (LH)
1.   M-C   Mouth to Crown (Caution, don't let hand touch the nose.)
2.   HT-C   Half way between Heart and Throat, to Crown
3.   SPH-C   Half way between Solar Plexus and Heart, to Crown
4.   KSP-C   Half way between Kath and Solar Plexus, to Crown
5.   PK-C   Half way between Pubic and Kath, to Crown
6.   RP-C   Half way between Root and Pubic, to Crown
7.   R-C   Root to Crown (LH stays at Crown, move RH to buttocks crease)
8.   Feet   RH on right foot and LH on left foot.

(Practical SHEN Sessions consist of three parts: 1. Relaxation (usually the Shoulder/Head Flows) 2. Opening up or releasing an emotion region and 3. Reintegration of the region with the rest of the field, usually Root and/or Crown Flows.

* * * * *

This completes the Lessons for Day 2. The following pages cover Outside Practice Sessions 3, 4, 5 and 6. You are to complete these in four weeksbut you may schedule them as often as two or three per week. (And you may do more than one of each.) **Outside Sessions 3, 4 and 5 need not be done in order, but Session 6 should be last.**

NOTE: It is much better to work with different partners during practice as all bodies will not respond the same or feel the same to you.

THIRD OUTSIDE PRACTICE SESSION   THE SOLAR PLEXUS
(You will need close to two hours if you both practice)

This session combines several types of flows, all focusing around the Solar Plexus. Work at this region is included in the SHEN protocols for poorly functioning digestive organs, with anorexia and with migraines that have an abdominal component. SHEN with anxiety, and the phobias is largely centered here. Spend enough time at each segment to feel a good strong effect

1. Shoulder/Head Flows
2. R-T
3. Right Side Peripheral, from Kath Line to Heart Line
4. Left Side Peripheral, from Kath Line to Heart Line
5. KSP^3
6. SPH^3
7. <SP>
8. SP^3
9. R-K
10. R-SP
11. KSP-C
12. R-C
13. Feet

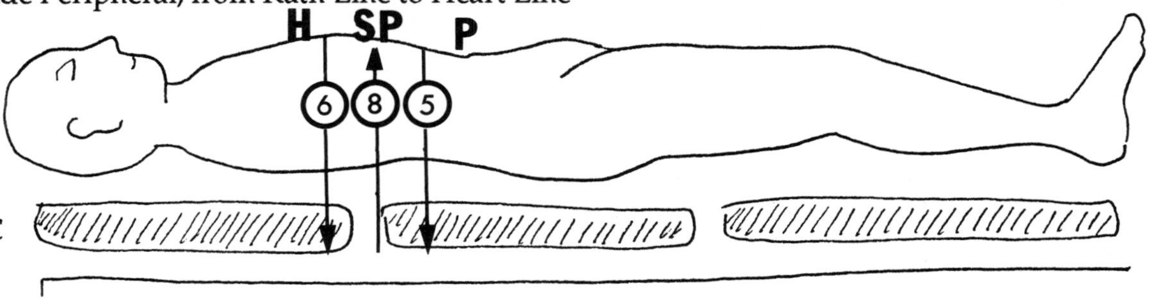

Figure 72 Solar Plexus Flows *(Supine)*

Observations about your session

Observations about the session you performed

Questions about these procedures

FOURTH OUTSIDE PRACTICE SESSION   THE HEART
(You will need close to two hours if you both practice)

This Session combines several flows around on the Heart Region. Work in this region is central to the SHEN protocols for migraine, high blood pressure, heart pain and SHEN work following heart attacks. SHEN for repressed grief is focused here.

1.   Shoulder/Head Flows
2.   R-T
3.   Right Side Peripheral, from Solar Plexus Line to Throat Line
4.   Left Side Peripheral, from Solar Plexus Line to Throat Line
5.   SPH^3
6.   HT^3
7.   <H>
8.   H^3
9.   SPH-C
10. R-K
11. R-H
12. R-C
13. Feet

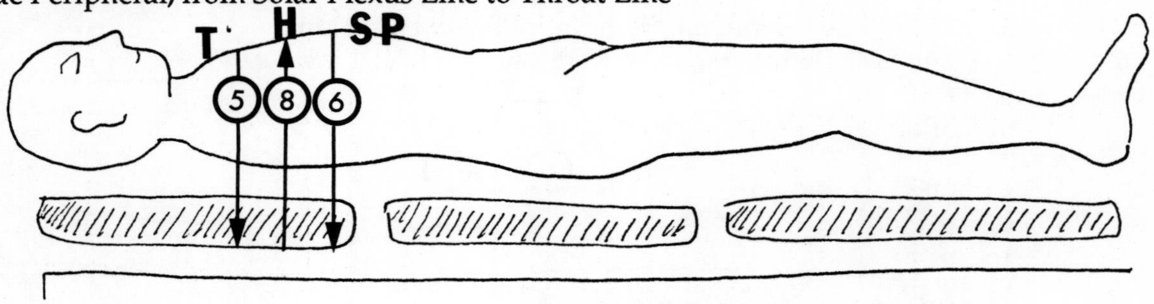

Figure 73 Heart Flows *(Supine)*

Observations about your session

Observations about the session you performed

Questions about these procedures

FIFTH OUTSIDE PRACTICE SESSION   THE PUBIC
(You will need nearly two hours if you both practice)

This session combines several flows around the Pubic Region. Work in this region is central to the SHEN protocols for excessive menstrual cramping, premenstrual distress and related syndromes. SHEN in this region has been quite helpful in aiding repressed sexual feeling.

1.   Shoulder/Head Flows
2.   R-T
3.   Right Side Peripheral, from Root Line to Kath Line
4.   Left Side Peripheral, from Root Line to Kath Line
5.   RP^3
6.   PK^3
7.   <P>
8.   P^3
9.   RP-C
10. R-P
11. R-K
12. R-C
13. Feet

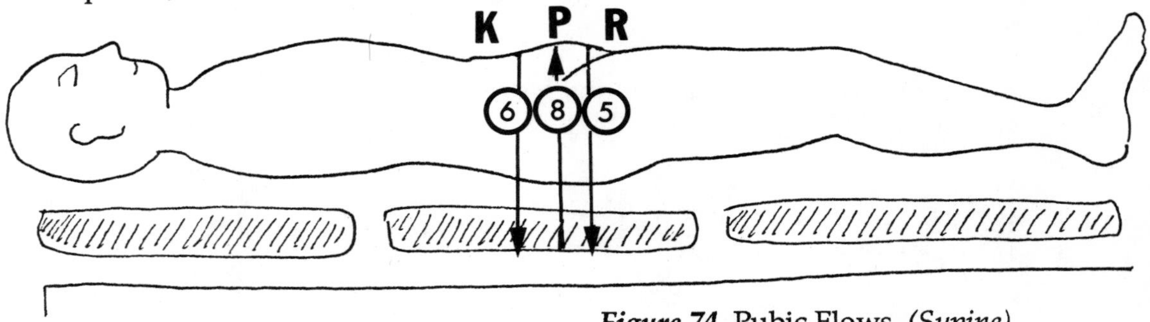

Figure 74 Pubic Flows *(Supine)*

Observations about your session

Observations about the session you performed

Questions about these procedures

SIXTH OUTSIDE PRACTICE SESSION   THE THROAT AND ROOT
(You will need just over two hours if you both practice)

SHEN work at the Throat has been helpful with chronic psychosomatic throat clearing and with lack of expressiveness. SHEN work at the Root figures heavily in work with the effects of rape, with night terrors and with post traumatic stress disorder.

1.   Shoulder/Head Flows
2.   R-T
3. M^2
4. HT^3
5.   HT-C
6.   <T>
7. T^3
8.   Right Side Peripheral, mid thigh to Kath Line
9.   Left Side Peripheral, mid thigh to Kath Line
10. RP^3
11. <R>
12. R
13. R-K
14. R-T
15. R-C
16. Feet

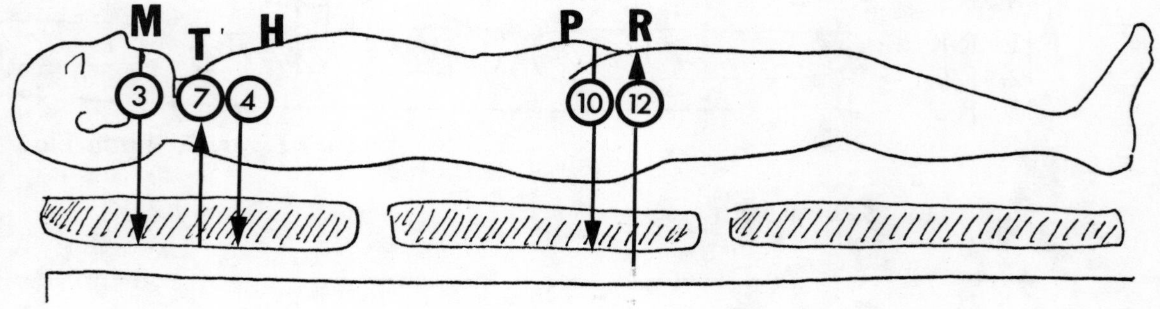

Figure 75 Throat Flows and Root Flows (*Supine*)

Observations about your session

Observations about session you did

Questions about these procedures

CHAPTER 11

ADVANCED SHEN PROCEDURES
(Training for Day Three of the Course.)

Refining Techniques. Much of your training so far has been intended to familiarize you with the anatomy of the Physioemotional Field. Today you will learn a number of ways to expand on the Flows you learned in Days 1 and 2 and how to combine parts of those flows in ways that are particularly useful in therapeutic work.

EXPANDING THE CROWN AND ROOT FLOWS.
When you learned the Crown and Root Flows you practiced them only on the midline. You can effectively expand these to the sides of the midline. The procedure works for all the regions but works especially well for the regions nearest the stationary hand.

EXPANDING THE ROOT FLOWS.
To do this, you place your Left Hand slightly off to one side or the other of the Midline, about where they would be when doing Triples. (Your Right Hand stays in the same place, at the Root.)

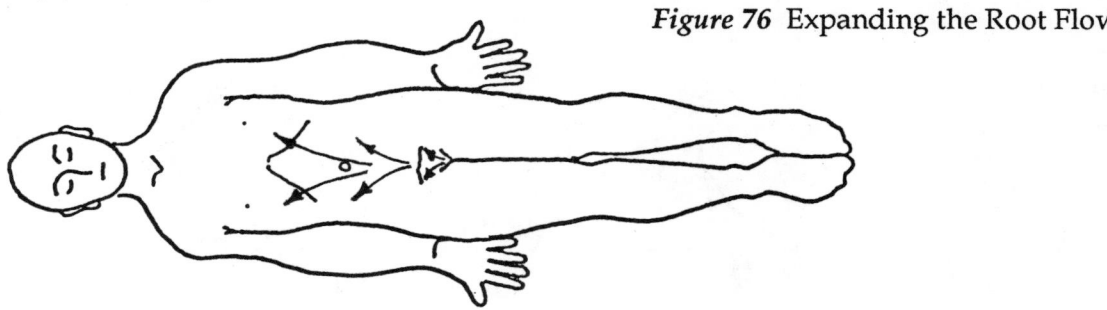

Figure 76 Expanding the Root Flows

Expanding the Crown Flows.
Place your Right Hand slightly off to either side of the midline between the Emotion Centers. (Your Left Hand stays in place at the Crown.)

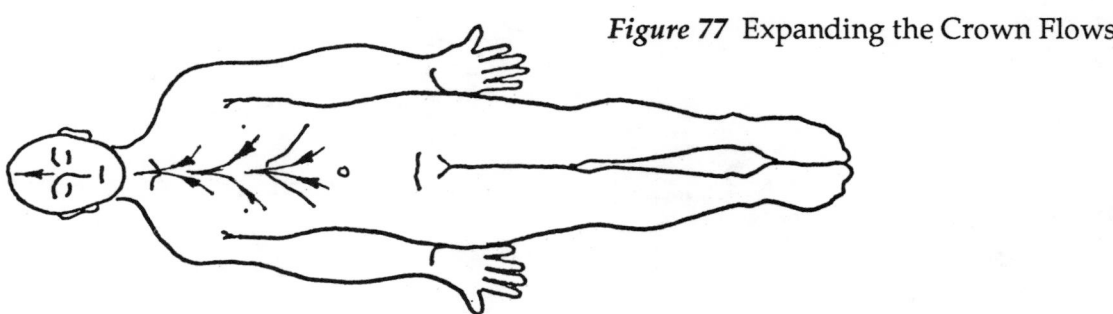

Figure 77 Expanding the Crown Flows

SHORTHAND NOTATIONS FOR EXPANDED ROOT AND CROWN FLOWS

Keeping notes is a simple extension of what you have already learned. Just put the superscript 3 following the notation you would ordinarily use for the Root or Crown Flows: $R\text{-}K^3$, $R\text{-}H^3$ or $SPH^3\text{-}C$, $HT^3\text{-}C$, etc.

FRONTAL FLOWS

Basically, the procedure is quite simple. Place your RH on a site in the body where the flow is moving inward (Rearward) and place your LH on a site where it is moves outward (Frontward). (Just be sure your hands don't touch each other.)

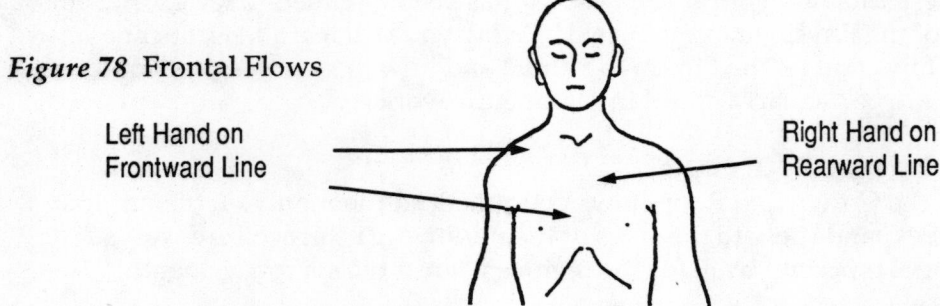

Figure 78 Frontal Flows

Left Hand on
Frontward Line

Right Hand on
Rearward Line

If you match the flows from your hands with the correct entry and exit sites, the flow you do will be carried deep into the body, if not the flow will merely skim the surface and not be effective.

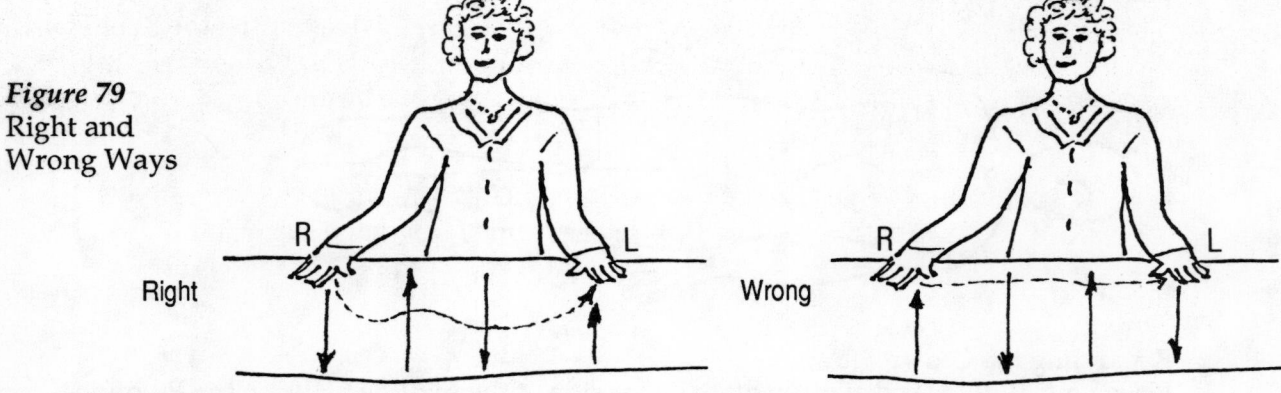

Figure 79
Right and
Wrong Ways

Right

Wrong

These flows can be done on either side, at the midline, or diagonally.

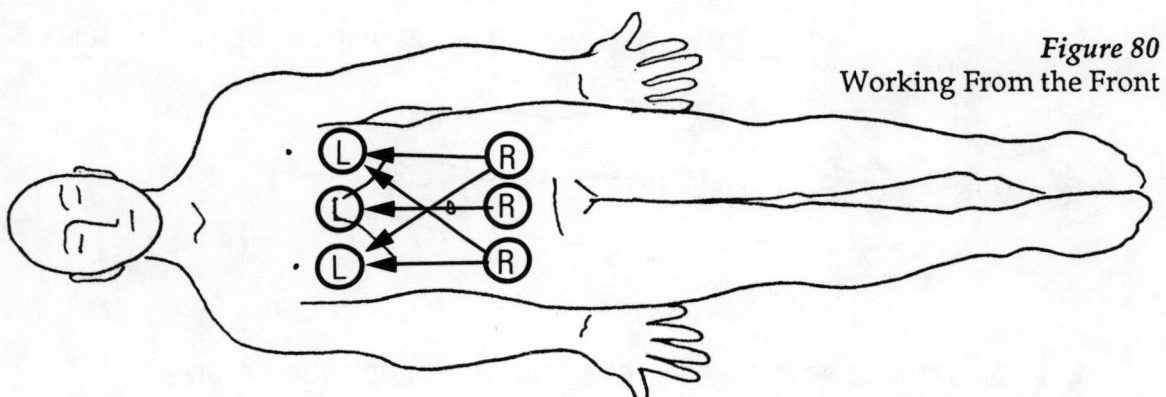

Figure 80
Working From the Front

NOTE: *When doing these flows, your hands are NOT as far out at the sides as they are when you do the Peripheral Flows.*

Frontal Flows can be directed towards either the head or the feet with this method. *(Since all of the flows are on the front of the body, none of them will interfere with the normal headward flow at the spine, nor with the peripheral movement.)* Downward Frontal Flows are very useful when the person has no energy at the Kath, when it is all at the Heart or Solar Plexus and they have difficulty functioning or being grounded.

Figure 81 Available Directions

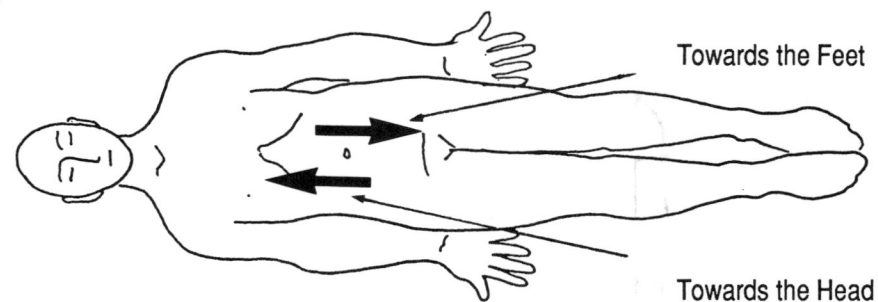

SHORTHAND NOTATIONS FOR THE FRONTAL FLOWS

The notations are probably obvious but I will spell them out anyway. Note the position of your RH, then a dash, then the position of your LH. (Your RH will always be on a rearward or inward flowing line, and your LH will always be on a frontward or outward flowing line.) RP^L-H^L, RP^L-H^R, KSP^R-T^R, KSP^R-T^L.

FIRST PRACTICE SESSION (DAY 3) EXPANDED ROOT, CROWN AND FRONTAL FLOWS
(Allow about an hour and a half if you both practice this)

Figure 82
First Session, Day 3

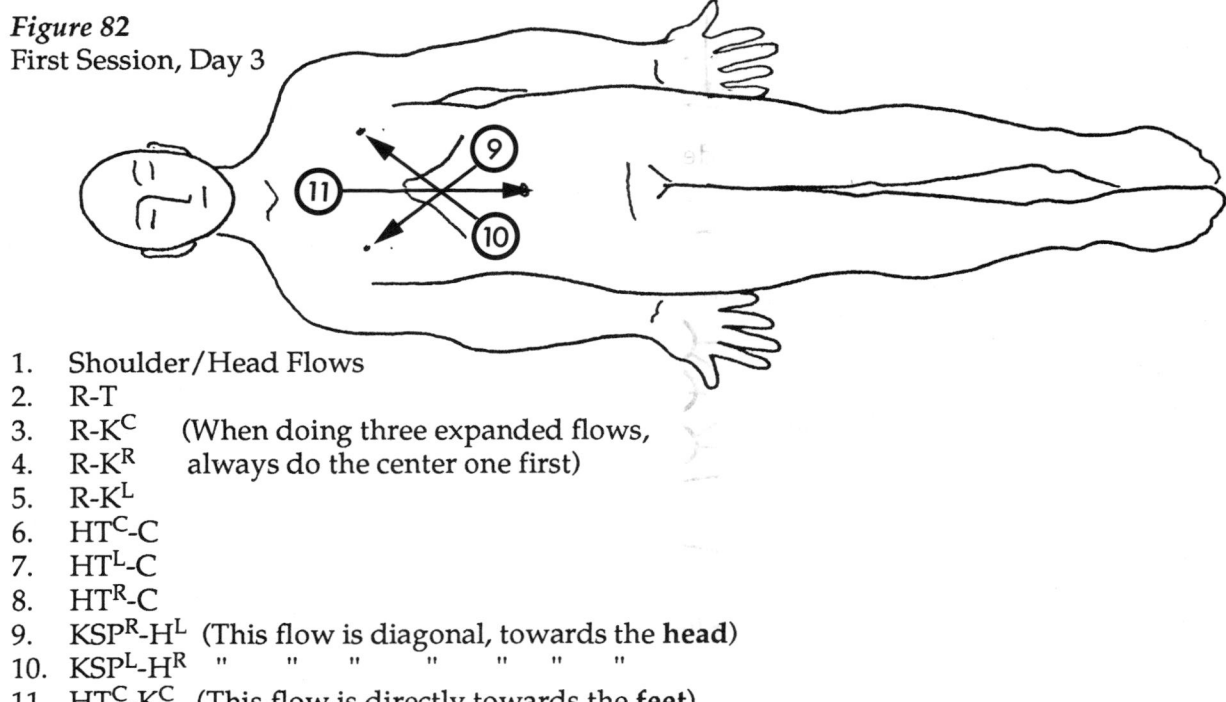

1. Shoulder/Head Flows
2. R-T
3. R-K^C (When doing three expanded flows,
4. R-K^R always do the center one first)
5. R-K^L
6. HT^C-C
7. HT^L-C
8. HT^R-C
9. KSP^R-H^L (This flow is diagonal, towards the **head**)
10. KSP^L-H^R "   "   "   "   "   "   "
11. HT^C-K^C (This flow is directly towards the **feet**)
12. R-C

FLOWS AT THE SIDES

These are quite simple, the hands are placed one above the other at the same emotion line or blocking segment. It is just like a triple except that the lower hand is brought out to the side, directly under its mate. As was explained before, you usually don't do this when doing triples to avoid disturbing the person but there are times when it is quite useful. (One of these is when working with irritable bowel syndrome, flows right through the ascending and descending colon are quite helpful.)

Figure 83
SHEN Flows
at the Sides

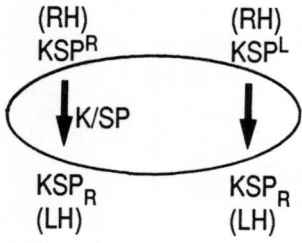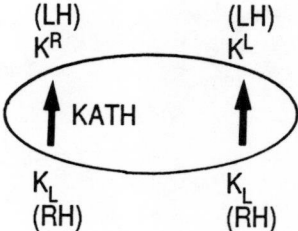

You can also do *diagonal* flows with your hands at the Sides. (Very useful with invalids when you can't get your hands under the spine.)

Figure 84
Diagonals
at the Sides

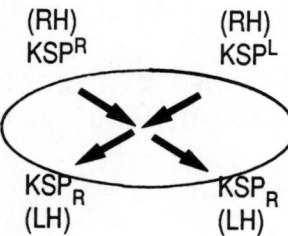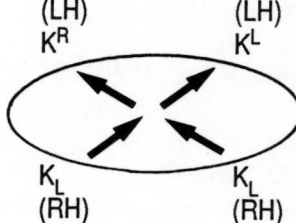

These procedures give you a number of ways to approach the regions or sectors that are deeply tense. You can work diagonally across a single region or you can use this method to promote emotional release at two emotion regions simultaneously.

There are times when it is useful to be able to do flows entirely from the front of the body. Some of these are:

(1) When the patient/client is injured or incapacitated and you can't get your hands under them in the way you normally would to do Frontward or Rearward Flows.

(2) When you would like to work with two of the emotion regions simultaneously in order to expedite the release process. Usually you would: a. Do Rearward Flows beside both emotion regions,

b.   Frontward Flows through both emotion regions and

c.   Frontal Flows from the far side of one emotion region to the other emotion region. Working with two emotion regions at once is quite useful when using SHEN for emotional release.

COMBINING FLOWS THROUGH TWO CENTERS

These flows are similar to the Root Flows. (When doing Root Flows your RH was **behind** one center (the Root) and your LH **on the front** of a different center. In the same fashion, you can put your RH behind **any** center and your LH on the front of **any other** center and do a flow that affects both centers but especially effects *the area between the centers.* You can do these as triples, if you wish.

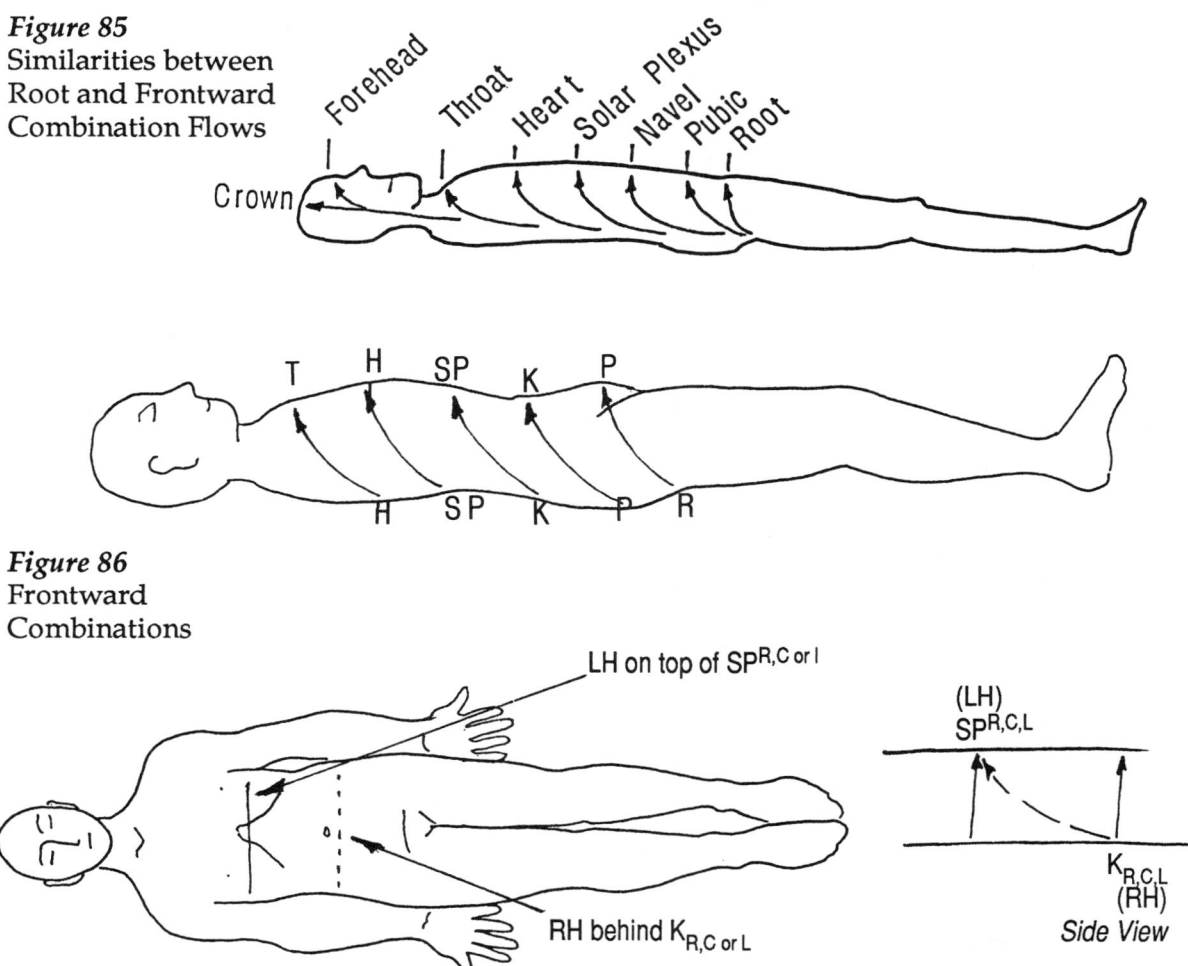

Figure 85
Similarities between Root and Frontward Combination Flows

Figure 86
Frontward Combinations

You can also do Rearward Combination Flows as well as Frontward Combination Flows. Rearward Combination Flows are similar to the Crown Flows. (See next page.)

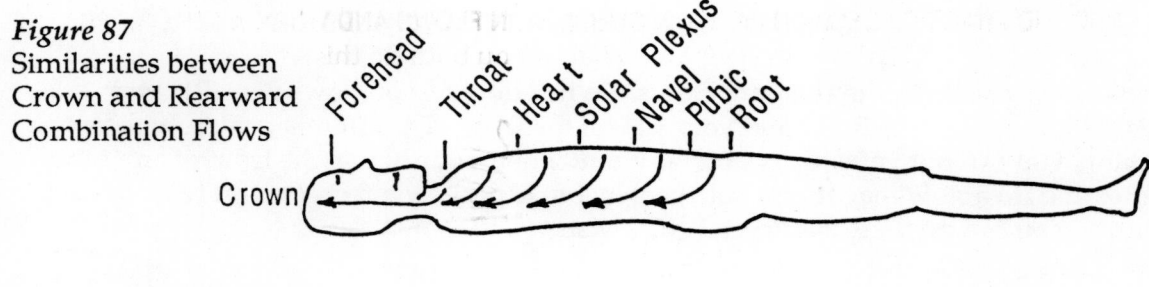

Figure 87
Similarities between
Crown and Rearward
Combination Flows

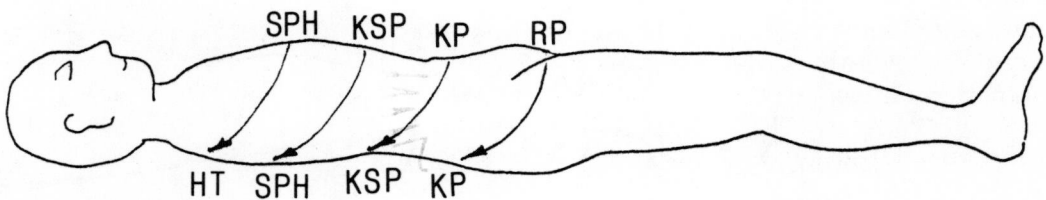

Figure 88
Rearward
Combinations

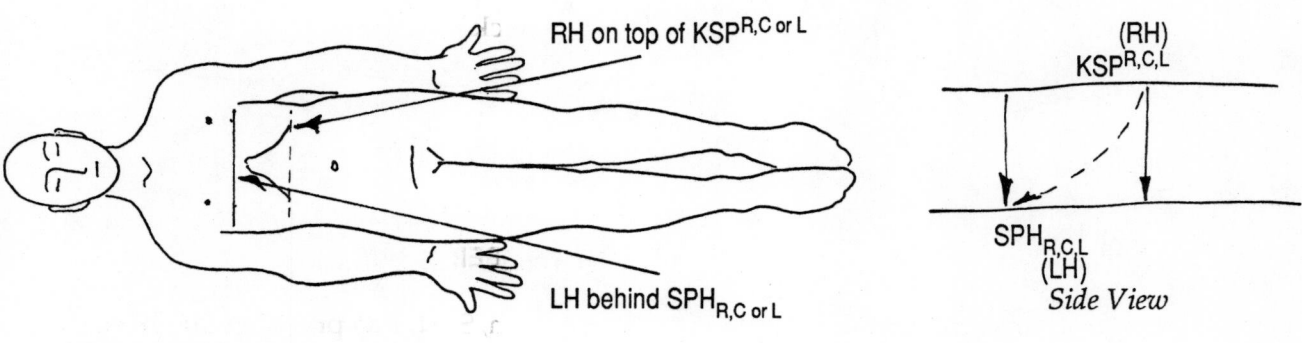

*NOTE: Either Frontward or Rearward Combination Flows can be done as **diagonal flows**, as well.* These can be very useful. For example, flows that go from the rear of the Pubic to the front of the Kath, and do it on a diagonal, move through the uterus. These flows are very useful with menstrual and premenstrual distress and when doing SHEN with rape victims. Similar diagonals through the body are used with other SHEN protocols.

Figure 89
Combination
Diagonals

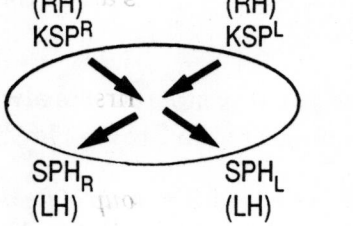
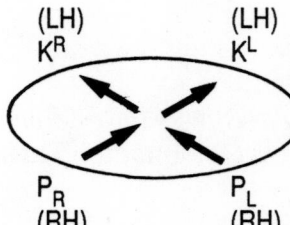

SECOND PRACTICE SESSION (DAY 3) COMBINATION FLOWS AND WORK AT THE SIDES

(Allow an hour and a half if you both do this)

Figure 90
Second Session
Day 3

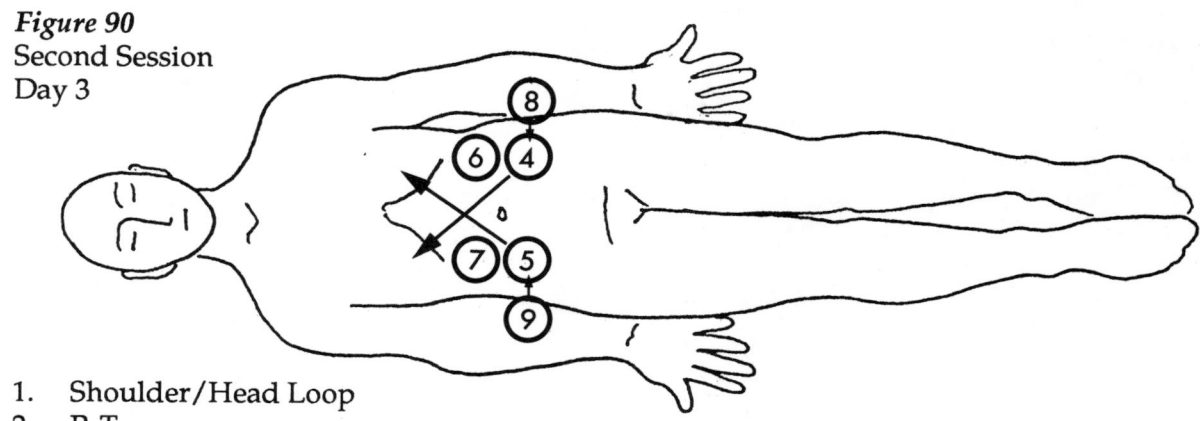

1. Shoulder/Head Loop
2. R-T
3. R-K^3
4. K_L-SP^R
5. K_R-SP^L
6. KSP^L-KSP_L (Careful, you need to switch hands from top to bottom.)
7. KSP^R-KSP_R
8. K_L-K^L (And now you need to switch back.)
9. K_R-K^R
10. R-K

* * * * *

POINTS TO REMEMBER

1. You can combine any pair of Lines (Heart, Kath, SPH, PK) provided that front or rearward movement is in the same direction through both.

2. You can work diagonally as well as vertically.

3. As long as your hands are on the *front* and not the sides or back, you can do flows that move in a downward direction.

4. It is best to have your lower hand next to the body and **not under** a cushion or mat. (For the Side Flows.) Since the lower hand positions are at the sides, rather than at the mid back, it should cause no discomfort.

5. In SHEN notations, the position that is written first is always your sending hand.

This completes the training. You have learned quite a group of flows with which you can work with a great many troublesome disorders quickly and efficiently. Now you can begin learning how to do therapeutic work with Shen.

REVIEW OF
CHAPTERS 10 AND 11

1. Identify the emotion regions

2. Indicate frontward and
    rearward movement

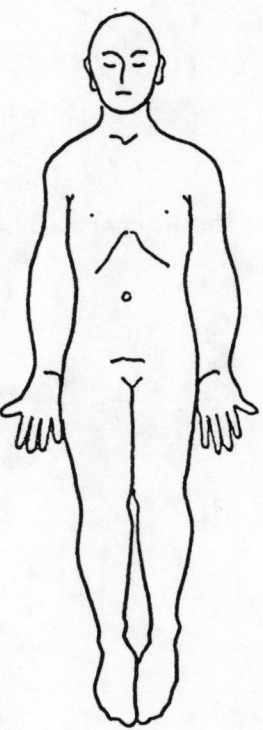

3. SPH refers to:

4. Reverse Flows:
    a. Are between the emotion centers.
    b. Are never done.
    c. Effectively clear blockages.

4. The two areas of greatest tension in the body are:
    a. Calves of the legs.
    b. The shoulders.
    c. The brain.
    d. The hands.

5. The Heart Center is located at:

6. The Kath is located at:

7. The Throat Center is located at:

8. The Root is located at the:

9. The Mouth is on a (Frontward) (Rearward) Line?

SHEN is more than just a science, it is an art.
Learning to use the tools is only the beginning.

CHAPTER 12   **SHEN SELF FLOWS** _____ *109*
        Doing SHEN on Yourself, 109.

CHAPTER 13   **PLANNING THE SESSION AND DEVELOPING THE TREATMENT SERIES** _____ *111*
        Planning the Session, 111. Developing the Treatment Series, 112. Scheduling, 112. Some Rules of
        Thumb, 113. Instructions to give the client, 114

CHAPTER 14   **COMBINING SHEN AND OTHER THERAPIES** _____ *115*
        Breathwork, Rebirthing, 115. Massage, 115. Imagery, 115. Gestalt, 116. Rolfing, 116.

CHAPTER 15   **SHEN THERAPY FOR EMOTIONAL AND PSYCHIATRIC DISORDERS** _____ *117*
        Major Depression, 117. Fear of Insanity, 118. Phobias, Anxiety Attacks, Patient in crisis, 118. Recurrent
        Images, Dreams, Nightmares, 119. Hallucinations, 119. General Considerations, 120. Children's Night
        Terrors, 121. Patient Management, 121.

CHAPTER 16   **EFFECTS OF SHEN ON THE "KUNDILINI CRISIS"** _____ *123*
        Pain During Meditation, 123. Ecstasy Turning to Pain, 124. Falling Out, 124. Kriyas, 125. Siddhas, 126.

CHAPTER 17   **SHEN IN THE HOSPITAL AND CLINIC** _____ *127*
        Panacea or Specific, 127. Swollen Tissue, 127. Pain, 127. Improving Organ Function, 128. Emotionally
        Influenced Disorders, 128. Physical Disorders with Emotional Results, 128. Emotionally Rooted Disorders,
        128. SHEN in the Hospital, 129. Pre & Post Surgery Procedures, 130. Psychogenic Shock, Some Coma,
        131. Fractures, Swollen and Sprained Joints, 131. Arthritis, 131. Bursitis, 131. Kidney Stones, 132.
        Gallstones, 132. Aches and Pains of the Aged, 132. Muscle Tension Headaches, 132. Sinus Headaches,
        132. Pregnancy and Birthing, 133. Vertigo, Tinnitus, 133. Jet Lag, 133. Protocols for Emotionally Rooted
        Disorders, 134. Irritable Bowel Syndrome, 134. Migraine and Migraine Variants, 135. Premenstrual and
        Menstrual Distress, 137. Anorexia/Eating Disorders, 138.

CHAPTER 18   **SHEN AND CHRONIC PAIN** _____ *139*
        Psychological Responses to Pain, 139. Major Pain Components in Chronic Pain Syndrome, 139.
        Development of Simple Chronic Pain, 140. Pre Injury Fear, 140. Post Injury Fear, 141. Non-Injury
        Related Emotional Components, 141. Emergence of Memory, 142. Development of Complex Chronic
        Pain, 142. Psychogenic Pain, 142. Chronic Low Back Syndrome, 144. Unremitting Psychogenic Pain
        Stemming From a Strong Blow, 145. Determining the Degree of Psychogenisity, 145. Expectations With
        Various Patients, 145. Patient Management and Concerns, 146.

Unless you learn to follow the signs that your patient/client presents, and to apply the SHEN techniques skillfully, you will have little to show for your effort. If you follow the procedures given you, you will never harm anyone, if you use inappropriate ones, you will not be effective.

CHAPTER 12

SHEN SELF FLOWS

Doing SHEN on Yourself

You can do a certain amount of SHEN work on yourself. It will not be quite as effective as having someone else work with you because then you have the fields from two of you focused at the problem and because you are limited as to the range of hand positions you can use, but there are ways to offset those drawbacks. And its worth it, SHEN work on yourself can be quite valuable.

ROOT FLOWS

If your arms are long enough you can slip your sending hand under your buttocks and place your receiving hand at any of the centers you choose to work with. You will need to prop your elbow up on a pillow so that it doesn't slip off as you drift out to sleep during the flow.

If your arms are too short to reach your buttocks, you can slip your hand under the small of your back (either palm up or palm down) and do flows through the upper centers. This position won't work on the lower centers very well. For them you can do:

TRANSVERSE FLOWS

It is quite easy to do transverse flows at the lower emotion regions and blocking segments, those from the Solar Plexus Line on down. You can just do the Heart Line and most can do the transverse SPH Line. And you can do the:

CROWN FLOWS

Doing Crown Flows is quite simple but you will need pillows wedged under your receiving hand to keep it at the Crown or it will slip down as the flow starts to come through. You can reach to do all the Crown Flows.

TRIPLE FLOWS

It is difficult to get your hand all the way under your body to your spine. However, you can do the diagonal flows and the side flows quite well. By combining these you can effectively cover the area that a triple would cover. For example, you could place your right hand at K_R and do K_R-K^L, K_R-K^C and K_R-K^R. And you can do PK^L-PK_L, PK^C-PK_L and PK^R-PK_L

ENHANCED BREATHING

Those of you who have done any of the various forms of breathwork (Rebirthing, etc.), will recognize this as a variation of those techniques. If you wish you can use the technique you are familiar with.

Once your hands are in place and supported and you have relaxed your throat, let your jaw drop slightly. Slowly begin to deepen your breathing, allowing your abdomen to fill as you fill your lungs with more and more air. Don't push the air out of your lungs at the end of a filling phase, let your chest and abdominal muscles relax so that the breath just falls out. Feel the tight places leave your lower abdomen as this happens - let your lower abdomen fill more and more, expanding into those formerly tight places.

This procedure causes the Field to move more rapidly through your body, energizing your emotion centers as well as your arms. This combination of enhancing effects works quite well. (For an explanation of why this works review Chapter 8, The Physioemotional Field and Physics.) *Don't expect to do more than one good flow before falling asleep.*

A plan I use myself is to do a different flow each night, working my way up (or down) the emotion centers. Sometimes not much happens but at other times there will be quite positive results, often with visual images. When I get an especially good result, I will go back to that center the next night. Perhaps, if I was doing a Root or Crown Flow I will do a Transverse at that line. (Or vice versa.)

THERAPEUTIC SELF FLOWS

SWOLLEN JOINTS
You can also do several therapeutic flows for yourself. You can do flows through a sprained or swollen knee or ankle, either transverse or in the normal flow direction for that limb. I broke the last migraine I ever had, several years ago, just as it was starting, with the Crown Flow HT-C.

LOW BACK PAIN
You can lie on your back, prop your knees up and do Transverse Flows through the region of low back pain. Try to do three, the first above, the second just below and the third right through the pain site.

GALLSTONES
It is possible to ease gallstone pain with Transverse Flows through the area of pain, you can also get one hand behind your back and the other on the front (be sure the flow is in the proper direction for that location.) I apparently had a stone pass while doing this once. There was a gurgle and suddenly the pain was gone. It didn't come back.

GETTING SET FOR THE BIG ONE
When that big scary project is looming up just in front of you, lie down, get comfortable and do a Transverse Flow through your Kath, enhancing your breath as you do it. Its great.

JET LAG
Do a Root to Crown Flow. Enhanced breathing will help.

DIZZINESS OR DISORIENTATION
Root to Crown with enhanced breathing.

CHAPTER 13

PLANNING THE SESSION AND DEVELOPING THE TREATMENT SERIES

PLANNING THE SESSION

READING THE SIGNS

Observe the client when they arrive. Notice their body posture, how do they look when they walk in, how do they sit, where do they put their hands - what are they guarding? What is their breathing like? Pay attention to the words they use, sometimes the real emotion, just below the surface, is masked by a conversation that is misleading. (Like when you automatically respond to the casual question "How are you?" with "Just fine!" when you are really feeling lousy.)

Before the session always ask about any emotion that may have emerged, unexpected memory (especially ask if it has new content) unusual dreams or changes in dream content that occurred since the last session. Changes in dreaming pattern indicate the emotions about to surface. Look for changes in color (are the dreams getting darker or lighter) are the nightmares not as frightening, etc.

After they lie down, notice where they place their hands, they may be guarding a painful center. Almost always the person will place their hands on the area that is painful, even though they are not aware of it. Notice their breath pattern. Is it in the chest, the lower belly, both? Is it biphasic, when the breath is still coming in at the belly just after the exhale starts at the chest? The fulcrum point is almost certainly a place of emotional pain. I have seen the location of the fulcrum shift during a single session as the emotional tensions changed.

Figure 91
Biphasic Breathing

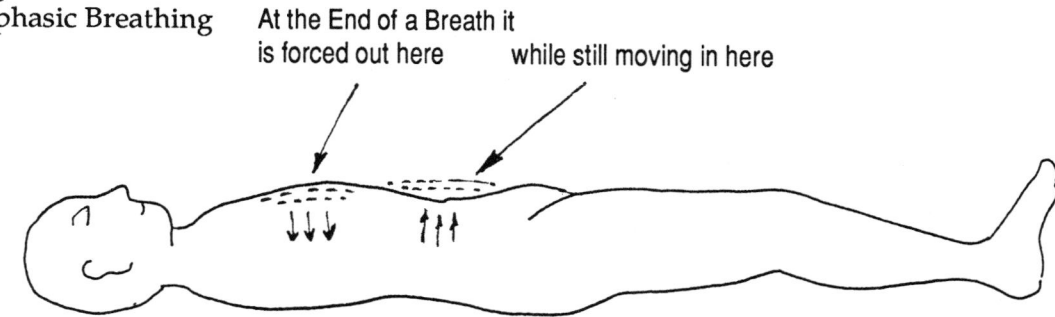

SCANNING WITH YOUR HAND

Pass the palm of you hand about an inch above the body, notice what you feel. The places where there is a noticeable shift in temperature sensation is likely to be a place of constriction. The change in temperature (if it is not due to differences in body fat) is due to differences in local tension. If you can't get an indication, try putting your right hand under the Root and pass your left hand over the body at a moderate rate while paying attention to the sensations in the palm of your *right hand (not your left hand)*.

Several different indicators (posture, breathing, hand scans), all pointing to the same location, will indicate a prime area for Shen.

DEVELOPING THE TREATMENT SERIES

SHEN FOR EMOTIONAL AWAKENING AND SELF REALIZATION

A good course of treatment to start out with is this:

Session 1: Full Peripheral Flows and ALL the Rearward Flows (No Frontward Flows) followed by R-K, R-C. This session begins to break all the contractile tension patterns in the torso. (With the depressed person you may need to repeat this session two or three times.)

Session 2: Relaxation Flows followed by work at the Kath Region. Kath work is first because we need to start accessing the buried feelings of confidence and adequacy as soon as possible. Work there keeps them grounded, together. If they start getting into fear, sexuality or sadness in the first session without being centered and without the beginnings of confidence, they may be overwhelmed by the experience and likely will not come back.

Session 3: Relaxation Flows followed by work at the Solar Plexus Region.

Session 4: Relaxation Flows followed by work at the Heart Region.

Session 5: Relaxation Flows followed by work at the Pubic Region.

Session 6: Relaxation Flows followed by work at the Root and Throat. Work at the Throat and Root is last because little happens at either place during the early sessions. (An exception is when the person is in the midst of a major transitional life change. Then Root work can be productive)

Session 7: Relaxation Flows, followed by work at the Kath and the Region that produced the major response.

This sequence is a guide only. You will probably change the order of these when you think it is appropriate. These sessions may uncover areas that need extra work. If so, you will want to repeat sessions where major releases occurred. People don't stand still when you do Shen. They move and they move fast. If you are not careful you will be left behind as they and their symptoms change. When they walk in the door expect them to be different than when you last saw them. The course you envision at the outset of a series will almost certainly be modified, if you are on your toes and observant of the client's changes.

SCHEDULING

EMOTIONAL AWAKENING

Sessions are best scheduled once or twice a week. More often than that will not give enough time to assimilate the material that may arise. Longer spacing will be less productive. With those who have emotional or psychiatric disorders closer scheduling is needed.

MAJOR DEPRESSION, ANXIETY ATTACKS, PHOBIAS, AND CHRONIC PSYCHOGENIC PAIN
Experience shows that these patients respond best to intensive SHEN. It is best to schedule these patients for daily sessions.

PSYCHOSOMATIC DISORDERS
These patients respond best to intensive, daily work during the high point of the trauma. The progress during treatment for emotionally derived disorders is not like progress with strictly biological illnesses. Once the regions involved with the original disorder begin to relax, other regions begin to open as well. The person suffering from an irritable bowel caused by retention of shame and inadequacy, for example, may later release sadness at the heart or fear at the solar plexus. You will have to work at these regions too.

SOME RULES OF THUMB

1. The larger the trauma the quicker and more dramatic the results. (Except for Major Depression where signs of progress will be small.)

2. When the emotion is buried, do Rearward Flows, when it emerges switch and do Frontward Flows. (This may come in the middle of a session.)

3. Your intention should be to assist the emergence of whatever occurs NOT to direct or pre-plan what YOU want to have happen.

4. Think of the session as having three parts: (A) Relaxation, usually shoulder/head flows, (B) the focus of the work at the region and (C) reintegration, usually with Root to Kath, Root to Crown, etc. Not doing this will leave them ungrounded and spacy.

5. When the client begins to bring up repressed emotion and memory, there is almost always need for counseling and direction. **If you are not a licensed pyschotherapist or counseler, be CERTAIN that the client has one.** It is best to have an open line of communication with that therapist.

6. Frequently work remote from the Solar Plexus brings up anxiety or fear. It is not necessary to switch locations and work at the Solar Plexus to accelerate it. Stay where you are, at least until it blossoms fully. If you move to the Solar Plexus you risk losing it while you transfer.

7. When sexual arousal comes up while working at the Pubic region, it may be frightening, sometimes because the feelings have never been experienced. This will have to be discussed from within the person's particular frame of reference.

8. The setting is important. It should have subdued lighting and be free from sudden noises. Use of a good ocean tape or record as background is desirable. Do NOT use music that evokes particular emotions. As soon as you try to program their emotions you lose the ability to access the emotions you are not aware of.

9. After the first session, explain that emotion may come up in dreaming or while awake during the next thirty-six hours, to let it happen, it needs to get out.

INSTRUCTIONS TO GIVE THE CLIENT

It is very frightening for some people to just "let go". Often this is because of unfamiliarity with the Shen Process, but it may be deeply ingrained because of past frights. The brain gets frightened when it is not busily being in charge. It is easy for them to decide to do any of a number of mental processes in order to "help". You need to emphasize:

Do not visualize yourself getting well. This is a good practice but it is counterproductive when done during SHEN because you cannot actively think and relax fully at the same time. Don't try to concentrate on anything, just let your mind float free, if thoughts come up notice them and let them go, don't dwell on them. If you drift off to sleep that's just fine.

The client/patient must understand that the statement "Emotion may come up" is literal and not figurative. Watch out for this one. Too often people say they are ready for emotion to come up but that doesn't mean that they expect to feel it. Tell them:

Emotion may come up, if it does that means you will feel it. For example, if anger comes up you will feel angry. This may (or may not) get intense. If it does get intense it will expand bigger and bigger then burst when the tension holding it is broken and dissipate rapidly. After it is gone that same anger will not return. And, it won't make you non-functioning while it happens.

Sometimes fear will come up. If you get afraid it may be easy to think that it is the Shen that is making you afraid. Just hang in there, if you do something will surface in your memory that will explain where the fear is really coming from. If you try to hold it back, it will stay inside and continue to trouble you. And, you are not likely to have the same experience twice in a row during the course of your Shen sessions.

DURING THE SESSION

When emotion emerges, and they cry or become frightened, be encouraging. Simple comments like "Good, Good" or "Unhuh!" A little touch of encouragement is all it takes in most cases. Don't just indicate that it is OK, say that it is good. Saying OK is neutral, indicating that it is desirable is much better.

CHAPTER 14

COMBINING SHEN AND OTHER THERAPIES

SHEN is an excellent adjunct to psychiatry and counselling, working to support those primary therapies, but no real combining of techniques is used. However with other therapies actual combining can be done successfully.

SHEN AND BREATHWORK - REBIRTHING.

This includes any of the amplified, exaggerated or otherwise accelerated guided breathing techniques used to promote the release of emotion and/or memory. (To understand how expanded breathing affects the Physioemotional Field, see Chapter 8, PHYSICS AND THE FIELD.)

The two systems are quite complementary. Breathwork works best with the Heart, Solar Plexus Regions. It has less effect with the Kath and much less with the Pubic and Root Regions. SHEN offsets this and gains from the breath amplified field.

It is quite simple to merge SHEN with breathwork. However, since the client needs to be instructed to keep the proper breath pattern going which probably means two therapists must be present. (It is extremely difficult to monitor and coach the breathing while doing flows.) When combining, do the flows exactly as you would normally do them. The amplification of the field adds to the total energy available and the therapist's hands serve to direct the amplified field to precisely the right spots.

SHEN AND MASSAGE

This combination is obvious. Interweaving SHEN and massage can be done at any point though you should pay attention to how relaxed the client is. If they fall asleep during SHEN you may not want to start digging into their muscles as it might disturb their relaxation. On the other hand this may be the time to get into areas that were like iron before.

I did a lot of this particular combination while taking a massage intensive many years ago. I did the SHEN after the massage and the combination was dynamite - emotion just poured out. Unfortunately, I never got my session, they were all limp as dishrags. Well, one must sacrifice for the good of science, I suppose!

SHEN AND IMAGERY

Specific Shen work at the cancer (or other disease) site frequently brings spontaneous images. If they come, these are prime images for the patient to work with. (Typically, with a patient that is healing, successive Shen sessions will bring images of lighter tone and with a color shift away from reds and blacks towards blues and greens.)

At any point the patient can creatively visualize these images changing toward more desirable ones. It is important, if further Shen at the site brings new and different images, that the old ones be discarded and the new ones used in the imaging process. Returning to old images will be counterproductive. If the imaging process works to heal, we can assume that working with older images would reverse the healing process.

SHEN AND GESTALT.

I am indebted for this process to my friend Charlotte McClure of Amarillo, Texas who developed it. Charlotte has her Gestalt clients half recline on a large bean-bag. She informs them that she intends to support them in their Gestalt dialogue and positions her hands to do a flow through the center she expects will be activated during the session. When the emotion begins, it just come flying out, in much greater volume than would be expected without the SHEN assist.

SHEN AND ROLFING™

Rolfing works on one side of the physical/emotional interface and Shen works on the other. The theories embraced by Rolfing are largely of the physical, the theories of Shen are largely of the physioemotional field or biofield. Nothing in Shen is contradictory to Rolfing perspectives. Shen procedures can assist the Rolfer in several ways:

1. When the client becomes overloaded: do the Peripheral segments which cross the region where you just finished working. Hold the flow for two or three minutes.

2. If there is a sudden emergence of grief, fear or shame do flows at the appropriate Emotion Region until the emerging emotion subsides. This will be brief. Following this the client should stabilize rapidly.

3. With specific body areas that are extremely sensitive to touch, Shen flows through that region before the deep tissue work will help:
   a. Do a transverse flow across the body at this area.
   b. Do Frontward or Rearward Flows appropriate to the area
   c. Finish with a peripheral flow through the region.

4. Specific muscle groups that are extremely bunched may be relaxed by doing flows along the length of the muscle group; your right hand at the point of insertion and your left hand at the point of origin.

5. If the client reports "feeling twisted" following a major rearrangement of musculature, have client move into the twist, i.e., accentuate the twist. Then do transverse flows *across the ends* of the twists.

6. If you do Shen flows after local tissue manipulation it is best to finish with a brief Peripheral Flow through the area.

7. Unlike deep tissue work Shen can be used directly at or on a trauma site where it is extremely effective in reducing pain and local edema. When working with pain, always place the hands so that flow carries the pain/emotion out of the body, not in to the body.

8. Following the Rolfing session:
   a. A brief flow through the region where the major work was done should help stabilize the client and prevent wild energy swings.
   b. A spinal flow (Root to Crown) can clear the head.

™ Rolfing is a Trade Mark of the Rolf Institute.

CHAPTER 15

SHEN THERAPY FOR EMOTIONAL AND PSYCHIATRIC DISORDERS

Shen can do much to support the psychiatrist's work by relieving secondary emotional complications and may occasionally contribute directly to treatment of the primary disorder.

At first thought one might be tempted to say, "Well, SHEN is OK for normals, (whoever *they* are) but not for psychiatric patients; after all, they are in serious trouble, perhaps with actual brain dysfunction." It seems to me to be worth remembering that underneath the psychiatric disorder is a real person, with real emotions. These emotions are sometimes a major part of the psychiatric problem and always color it to some degree. Indeed, one emotion, fear, frequently plays a major part in the course of treatment. This particular fear is usually unspoken and prevents the patient from cooperating in their treatment. It is the fear of insanityand is a complicating factor that the psychiatrist could well do without.

MAJOR DEPRESSION
(SHEN will not be very effective if cause is genetic.) Inherent in this disorder is the long term repression of all the emotions and their associated somatic affects. Occasionally a patient with virtually no muscle tone will complain of feeling tension "all over" their body. This is indicative of the deep constriction of the somatic affect. "Scanning" the body will detect little or no energy.

Spacing the sessions once a day may be the only way to crack the depression. If you space the sessions at longer intervals, the contractile tensions will be re-established, and you will make little progress.

Plan to do nothing but Rearward Flows for the first two sessions or so. This will begin to open up the contractile tensions. (If you see emotion beginning to surface during one of them, by all means follow it with appropriate Frontward Flows.) By the time you are into the third some cracks in the armor should be appearing that you can use to advantage. Sometimes the presence of superficial pain suggests an entry point for the series. Close attention to breath patterns may reveal the chink in the armor most susceptible to treatment.

(**Caution:** Don't assume the depressed patient is stuck merely because the patient does not give large colorful descriptions. The depressive will progress in the same steps as the normal person but since he/she is not emotive, the color and breadth of what is reported is reduced. Inability to express is not a sign of lack of progress. Don't become stuck at the place where the patient was, after he/she has moved on.)

At some point during the course of treatment the patient will likely report becoming "anxious" or "nervous". This is the indication that some emotion is about to surface. The emerging emotion may come from any center but causes nervousness because the feeling of any emotion is frightening to the depressed patient. *(This may prompt the patient to try to halt the SHEN series.)* Flows at the center that produced this effect should be alternated with flows at the Solar Plexus.

Eventually the anxiety will become identifiable as fear and this may be followed by a jumble of poorly defined emotions, prompting complaints of stomach discomfort and uneasiness. (At this point the Shen therapist is likely to match the patient by becoming puzzled and confused also. The patient is likely to say, "I don't know what it all means". This is a good time to be "real" and tell the patient that you don't know what the jumble means either right now, but it will soon be clear. Explain that what is happening is the first step of release of emotions, and that as the jumble subsides it will be replaced by definable emotions of longer duration, usually connected with clearer thoughts.

Frontward flows at Root and at Throat are appropriate. Flows at Root will usually not produce much result until the third or fourth session. Flows at Throat should be done as soon as the patient begins to struggle with expressing either verbally or through physical movement. **Note**: Progress is often (but not always) slow and it is easy to be tempted to abandon your efforts.

Patient "A", suffering from major depression. Within ten days (four SHEN treatments) "A" went from a monosyllabic conversationalist with absolutely flat affect and no interest in life's activities to one who smiled, giggled, expressed a little anger when appropriate, had begun recalling and recording her dreams (for the first time) and had started reading a book, "On how to improve your life". (She pointed out that it had been written by a woman.) She had been hospitalized for three months without any noticeable progress, it was her third hospitalization.

FEAR OF INSANITY

Often the fear of being insane is a big factor that must be overcome before treatment can be effective. The patient deeply afraid of insanity will be in denial of his or her condition. This particular fear is difficult to dislodge because its somatic affect is coupled with related fears under a common blanket of restriction covering the Kath and the Solar Plexus. Shen work at the Solar Plexus and Kath can elevate this particular fear, which is usually current and fairly superficial, often dissipating it in one or two sessions. Follow with more work at the Kath. Flows at root are appropriate. Once the patient is out of denial, the psychiatrists job will be much easier.

Patient "B", hospitalized for schizophrenia with auditory hallucinations was given her first SHEN treatment following which she asked the SHEN therapist, "Did you feel that motion at my stomach?" (Indicating her Kath/Solar Plexus Region). "That was when I gave up my fear of insanity". Her concern about being insane that had been interfering with her treatment was never again evident. And her confidence increased markedly following that treatment.

PHOBIAS, ANXIETY ATTACKS, PATIENT IN CRISIS

Little work is needed at the blocking segments to unlock the emotions as they are bursting to get out; there is little resistance to be broken. Work with the appropriate region can be started in the first session. (Use this approach with all those who have a great deal of emotion lurking just below the surface.)

RECURRENT IMAGES, DREAMS AND NIGHTMARES

Recurrent images of these sorts are evidence of some emotional process that is stuck. The approach with SHEN is to accelerate the patient out of their "stuckness". In order to determine a treatment plan, accept the recurring images as metaphor of some real emotional condition and perform treatments as you would if the events depicted were real. Evaluate the injuries or trauma in the nightmare and determine the emotions that would result if they were real and proceed accordingly. Often patients receiving SHEN treatments report improved sleep patterns, more vivid dreaming and a shift in dream content away from nightmares toward more pleasant dreaming. (There are examples of working with metaphorical images in the chapter of SHEN AND CHRONIC PAIN.)

Patient "C", hospitalized for psychotic depression with alcoholism. Following a SHEN treatment his dreaming increased from practically none. He experienced a vivid dream in which he was in a corridor with many doors. He opened each in turn only to find all the doorways bricked up. Soon after a second treatment, around his solar plexus, his anxiety elevated to where he became noticeably agitated. Shortly he recalled a job related incident thirty years before while in the Army that had troubled him deeply. (He had been ordered to do something which he considered to be unethical). As the emotion surfaced and completed the agitation ended. Two days later the dream repeated but now none of the doorways were bricked up. His anxiety did not return and he began to experience confidence that he would get well. His improvement continued and shortly afterwards he was discharged.

HALLUCINATIONS

Some studies indicate that auditory or visual hallucinations occur to perhaps twenty-five percent of the population. Whether the person needs psychiatric treatment for this condition is largely determined by the patient's sense of self. If the person has a good sense of self he or she is likely to treat the event as unexplainable but non-threatening and will not be influenced by the voices.

However, the person who is needy in the area of self-worth will respond differently. They will either become awed (frightened) by the voices and interpret them as threatening (evil spirits, the Devil) or will embrace the voices as allies (friendly guides, God) and convert their awe into personal specialness and use it as an antidote for their inadequate sense of self-worth.

SHEN treatment in these cases is to assist the emergence of feelings of self worth by doing flows at Kath and at Solar Plexus. The fearful patient becomes less fearful and as strength of self improves the voices begin to become less threatening and eventually recede, often entirely.

The patient who was frightened loses their fear and the one made "special" becomes less attached, less needful of the voices so they are likely to stop speaking as often. (Sometimes the "voices" tell the patient not to have any more Shen, just as if they were afraid of losing control over the patient.)

Enhancing the patient's sense of basic worth can be of considerable benefit to the psychiatrist. The presence of strong voices will draw the patient into their circle of influence and away from the influence of the psychiatrist. As the voices become weaker their influence is weaker and the patient becomes less antagonistic to treatment.

GENERAL CONSIDERATIONS - WORKING WITH THE PSYCHIATRIC PATIENT

The psychiatric patient seems to understand visceral concepts of emotion quite well. Concepts such as, "SHEN releases the emotions that are stuck in the body making you sick", or, "SHEN can bring the emotions up where you feel them - then you can finish them so they will go away and leave you alone" seem to be well received and understood. Explanations along this line give you a firm working base. Presenting SHEN innocuously often backfires. He/she will soon discover that much more happens then just "better rest" and "feeling better". If you haven't warned them they will resist later treatment.

It is extremely important when doing SHEN with psychiatric patients to be as direct and real as possible. If realness cannot be established the patient will not feel safe in revealing the material that arises during the session. Remember that this patient, more so than any other person you will work with, is in a constant defensive posture around his or her feelings of self worth and sense of security.

SHEN shakes that fragile, tenuous security. You are attempting to lead the patient into the deepest of his or her "scary places", places they try hard to avoid. You cannot lead them there if they do not have complete trust in you. If they try to fake you out about something, don't buy into it when you know they are hiding something - or THEY won't trust YOU. If you see physical responses that tell you something emotional happened during the session and they later tell you "Nothing happened" smile and say "Didn't I see some anger? (or whatever) when I had may hand at ___." They will likely agree but in any event will know they can't fake you, that it's time to be real. If you get angry at their reticence, their attempts to fake it, tell them so. "How can I help you when you won't let me?", tells them exactly where the two of you are.

Show yourself if you expect them to show themselves. When you don't understand what some memory or image means, say so. Explain that more information will come out in later sessions, that confused jumbled pictures, thoughts and words are the first things that come out as the emotions hidden inside are released. Don't expect the patient to be able to focus much at this stage.

"What does that mean to you" is not always a good question. They have difficulty enough in trying to understand. It is better to ask a range of questions designed to expand the amount of information. Simple, innocuous questions such as "What color was that" "Was it big" "What else was there" can help expand their memory and may trigger additional information. Expand their statements about their condition, too. If they say "I am in pain" ask: "Physical or emotional?" After they answer you can ask "where in the body".

Remember **"It's hopeless"** really means **"I am hopeless, powerless"**. This may be the first indication of emotion to emerge or be emphasized when work begins at the Kath. It is the upper or dominant feeling at that center. Keep going, later work will bring better memories and feelings, the beginnings of confidence, etc.

SHEN TREATMENT PROTOCOL   **CHILDREN'S NIGHT TERRORS**

1. Flow at Root (back to front)
2. Root to Kath
3. Root to Crown

(You can teach children to do a flow though their own Kath if they get afraid at night. Kids can sense the energy between their hands quite well. Have them find the place where they sense the tingles between their hands and then rotate their hands until it is strong. Then have them place their hands at their sides, in line with their belly button and keep them there until they feel the tingles through their tummies. They will often fall asleep in the middle.)

PATIENT MANAGEMENT CONSIDERATIONS

There are no special concerns or management requirements and there are no known adverse reactions or contra-indications. The emergence of emotion needs to be followed carefully as it will likely surprise the patient.

The improvement of sleep will benefit most patients. It is reasonable to expect fewer requests for sleep medications.

CHAPTER 16

EFFECTS OF SHEN ON THE "KUNDALINI CRISIS"

This experience is one of a type classified as *Spiritual Emergence* that can take many forms but most involve the manifestation of extreme energy movements in the body. The word *Kundalini* is taken from the Hindu, where the phenomenon called *Awakening of the Serpent Power* has been investigated and accepted for some time. The effects of the rise of Kundalini are called *Kriyas* and manifest as powerful sensations of energy or heat moving up the spine and may include tremors, violent shaking and twisted postures. The episodes often begin following an intense meditation practice that is not guided by a knowledgeable leader. (Variations of this crisis have occurred to followers of all spiritual disciplines.)

Intense pain can accompany the Kriyas and the episodes may include involuntary laughing, crying, talking in tongues, or other vocal noises. Psychic openings may occur that include the full range of parapsychological experiences. These experiences may flood in at a bewildering rate.

The most important thing is getting a useful perspective. The more you think of this situation as being untouchable because it is spiritual, and therefore unknowable, the less you will be able to help. And there is much you can do with SHEN that can help.

The usual approach is through counseling of a specialized but supportive nature. SHEN will complement that approach by providing relief from the grosser symptoms of physical pain and relief from fear and confusion.

The core of the phenomenon is in the energy field. When you view the process as a *flow of energy that gets blocked* you can immediately see how SHEN can be used to provide relief. The following cases illustrate various presentations of the Kundalini Crisis and the results of SHEN.

PAIN DURING MEDITATION.

"S" had increased his meditation practice for about a year until he began having intense abdominal heat while he meditated. If he did not break off the meditation the ball of heat would, "Suddenly jump to my head and become a severe headache". He was referred to me by a psychiatrist with considerable expertise in the field.

I agreed to work with S during one of his episodes, if we could time it right. A few days later he called to advise that one was beginning. I was free so he rushed over to see me and arrived with the intense heat still in his abdomen.

A very short (ten minute) session at the region between Kath and Solar Plexus released the heat and caused him to drop into a very deep state with quite pronounced REM. When he roused after the session he reported having two past life recalls flash by. He identified one as being in China. He did not get a headache.

He never again had the heat buildup or the headache during meditation.

ECSTASY TURNING INTO PAIN

"W" was a Rajneesh Sanyasin. Each time she would visit Rajneeshpuram or Poona she would become filled with ecstasy for several days until the ecstatic state would end with a crash, leaving her with head and stomach pains. She became so sensitive that this would occur if she would have a massage or if any kind of energy work was done to her.

The first SHEN session was performed largely around her heart. She began moaning, her tongue lolling about, salivating and her eyes rolled back, drool bubbled from her mouth as she began babylike cooing. Later she reported that these were involuntary, she had no control over them. These symptoms began as the flows started and continued until just after they stopped. They subsided without the usual head pain, perhaps because the event hadn't been sustained long enough. It seemed that all the energy was concentrating in the Heart Region, with none at the Kath.

Second session. I decided to short circuit the process and see what would happen if I didn't work at her heart. I began working between the Kath and Solar Plexus and then moved to the Kath. She dropped into a deep hypnogogic state rapidly with multiple episodes of REM and myoclonic jerks. None of the ecstatic phenomena occurred. She reported having had many, many "dreams" but could not recall their content.

Failed to come for another session. Reported that she no longer had the head and body pain following the ecstatic events but she had elected to discontinue the SHEN because her goal had been to extend the ecstasy indefinitely. (It helps if you and your client have the same goals.)

FALLING OUT

"J" fell out while singing in a gospel choir. Often singers fall out, lying on the floor in a state of ecstasy for some time. Falling out occurs frequently with gospel singers who adopt a particular breathing style. The breath is forced, almost pumped out so the the words come out in a forced almost staccato manner. Large volumes of air are inhaled and exhaled in this exaggerated fashion. Most of this breath movement was in the upper torso. It is easy to see what effect this would have on the physioemotional field. The Heart Region would be filled and expanded but the Kath, the center of balance, would not.

The experience is considered to be spiritual because it produces strong heart sensations and because of the lyrics. (The same experience would occur regardless of the lyrics.) Those who fall out, literally fall to the ground, unable to stand and consider themselves to be blessed by the experience. Some sing just for the possibility of having the experience.

I happened to be present during the gospel choir's presentation when this happened to J. As the service ended, she did not move but made tiny hand motions to get me to approach. She had difficulty talking and she looked about to faint. (Later she told me she had locked her knees or she would have fallen right there.) I half carried her into the pastor's study and laid her on the floor and did SHEN Flows through the Kath until she revived and was grounded enough to drive home. (She gave up the gospel singing on the grounds that it took too much out of her.)

SIDDHAS

"L" began having "spontaneous siddhas" after a year of practicing Transcendental Meditation fairly heavily. (Siddhas is an inclusive term for Kriyas and associated psychic events.) Internal shaking, pains in head and body, extreme rushes of fear and anxiety. Heard weird voices frequently. When she dances she expects the symptoms to reoccur if they have been dormant.

Every night feels like she has fallen into a hole and has to run. Is now eating red meat in the hopes that it will help her stabilize. Thought she had a heart attack a week ago. Her meditation teacher abandoned her "Because he didn't know what to do."

One session. The fear and anxiety elevated radically while the session was going on. She tried to fight against the experience, and so remained stuck in it. Agreed to come for a second session but canceled because she "Didn't want to feel the fear". Elected to give up dancing and her vegetarian diet in the hope that it would help.

It is not uncommon for dancing to aggravate these experiences, especially free-ranging, expansive dancing.

KRIYAS

"D" (Case Notes) History: Trained in Shen. Events during Shen sessions included remembrance and release of several past life traumas, fear, anxiety and beginnings of emergence of self confidence.

Kryia Event: Pains in abdomen, "weird energy": Body moving back and forth, "Spine tenses and pushes me into these postures". These incidents are occurring in association with "incredible meditations". Going into spontaneous meditations - "Roommates would walk by - I would not be affected. My body would go into a pulse, I would feel very secure, lot of gold light, energy flowing in - laughing - knew roommates observing but she didn't care. After the spontaneous meditation - big smile, began dancing round the room.

That night - real extreme reaction: Real tight feeling in abdomen while attending a concert. Later, lying down, "body began shaking (whole body trembling), got really cold. Abdomen knotted at Solar Plexus and Kath simultaneously, doubled over because it hurt so much , cried a little bit, breathed a little bit and then it pushed into my back and then my head would arch back and then go forward." The cycles repeated for about 45 minutes. Then stopped abruptly. "Felt really soft after that and I fell asleep." Slept all night woke refreshed. "D" reports no alcohol or grass or other stimulant during concert. (Does not indulge.) Not aware of grass in the vicinity.

Session two days after the incident. Started with flow up spine, Root to Crown. Shortly began to have pain - she pointed to Solar Plexus , shivering, body heat elevated. Periods of breath rate change but not enough to hyperventilate, periods of sobbing, "I just want the pain to stop". Contractions between Kath and Solar Plexus in cycles. Ended session when she expressed that she just wanted it to stop for a while.

Sat up, drank a sip of water, lay face down - sobbed briefly - "Feeling the despair I felt as a little kid.... legs feel nice and warm ... had a lot more energy in my legs lately - I usually [for a large part of life] didn't feel them.... lot of shooting energy up my legs last week... I'm reowning them". At this point she got up. Looked OK - reports feeling pretty good but a little shaky.

Later event: In meditation for four hours. Began to expand the pain and then became separate from it. "Learning to deal with the pain better, Still at the Kath and Solar Plexus. Third eye feels wide open - psychic vision has been going on for a long time. There is pressure at that spot." Bad events occur "When I call them" (Such as) "Branches fall, cars stop, the electricity goes out."

Session: Did KSP^3 Flows. Eyes flickered and got still. R-K strong and R-SP, strong. Little trauma this time. Later she asked if we could get together and talk (First time that she has not merely focussed on her problem.)

CHAPTER 17

SHEN IN THE HOSPITAL AND CLINIC

PANACEA OR SPECIFIC?
It is easy, too easy, when a new therapeutic tool is discovered to assign it near magical powers; the ability to affect an impossibly wide spectrum of ailments. It is hard to resist the temptation of thinking that it will be of value with anything and everything just because it does exceedingly well with some disorders. This is especially true of SHEN, not only because it can and does produce extremely good, sometimes startling, results with a number of seemingly diverse disorders, but because the idea of merely putting your hands on someone who is ill and "curing" them smacks of the magical. Invariably, those who do overreach, and attempt to use SHEN with inappropriate disorders, are caught up short when they discover that it is ineffective with those disorders.

This is the point where those who studied and grasped the theoretical background of SHEN are separated from those who did not. Those who failed to grasp its roots become dismayed and unsure of using it in the future, thinking that it has failed; those who understand its limitations will realize that SHEN did not fail, that it never would perform in those cases because it was an inappropriate therapy.

SHEN has only small effect on viral or bacterial diseases. It does not directly destroy viral or bacterial agents. Whatever effects are obtained with these diseases are through relaxation of fear, improved circulation, appetite and breath. All of these results contribute to the body's defense by assisting the immune system. (SHEN at the thymus often helps the immune system.) And the lessening of bodily sensations for a while will certainly be of help.

SHEN does several things well, all stemming from one central ability - the ability to cause extremely deep relaxation of local body tissue and to do this to a depth not possible with other methods.

SWOLLEN TISSUE
SHEN reduces local swelling by releasing the tensions surrounding the site of swelling. With local tension lowered, swelling reduces. The bloated tissue is drained of the stagnant fluid that is filled with waste metabolites. This accelerates the healing process because, with the mass of waste metabolic residue removed, the region is able to receive and utilize fresh supplies of hemoglobin, white blood cells, et al. *This is analogous to the closet that is stuffed full of junk - you can't put anything into it until you clean it out.*

PAIN
SHEN relaxes local tension in the body that, while perhaps started consciously, has become imbedded in the subconscious command structure and cannot be dislodged by mental processes. Thus SHEN has major application in treatment of psychogenic pain, the unexplainable pain surrounding old but biologically healed wounds. While it may reduce the tensional pain around a current injury, SHEN will not eliminate the pain normally generated by the biological healing process, the pain that signals us to care for that injury.

127

IMPROVING ORGAN FUNCTION

If tension caused by emotional pain surrounds organs in the body they will not function properly. The functioning, or manufacturing, cells of all organs and glands cannot function effectively when surrounded by stagnant, waste metabolites. Accumulation of waste metabolites interferes with the delivery of oxygen and other nutrients and prevent the outflow of future waste. Thus, the angry passive-aggressive anorectic's digestive shutdown is caused **in part** by the tension surrounding the digestive organs. Obviously, SHEN will help with this patient. And with the ulcer-prone patient. But not, for example, with a purely genetic pancreatic disorder.

EMOTIONALLY INFLUENCED DISORDERS

That emotion is intertwined with most physical disorders and can effect their outcome is rarely questioned. There are two basic types of emotionally influenced disorders, those where the emotion was caused by the disorder, and those where the emotion itself caused the disorder. SHEN is effective with either, but different approaches are taken with the two types.

PHYSICAL DISORDERS WITH EMOTIONAL RESULTS

The site of physical disorder and the site of the region of emotional response to that disorder are not always the same. A person who breaks a leg while falling down a flight of stairs may suffer from symptoms of loss of appetite, shortness of breath and reduced adrenal function. These symptoms are the result of fear retained at the Solar Plexus. The repression impacts on the biological functioning of the pancreas, adrenals, duodenum and diaphragm.

Many people in this situation have released fear following SHEN work and this has been followed in turn by increased appetite, improved breath intake and an improved outlook on life. If the fear was intense and included fear of death, contractile tension may still be in place at the Root. This will cause a general shutdown and depression. This needs to be taken into consideration. If the patient says things like "Well, I'm not as young as I used to be, I shouldn't be taking risks like that" and if their activity level is lower than before the trauma occurred, SHEN at the Root may change their outlook.

If SHEN is to be used to maximum effectiveness, the therapist will need to address those symptoms in designing a treatment plan. Simply using SHEN flows around the site of a broken leg is not enough.

EMOTIONALLY ROOTED DISORDERS. Here is where SHEN gets high marks. These disorders are caused by the imbedding of emotion in the body through repression of painful somatic affect in body regions encompassing organs and glands. Releasing the long-forgotten emotion ends the need to repress the painful somatic affect that accompanies it. Breaking the contractile tensions that affect the disfunctioning organs allows them to begin functioning normally. But don't overlook other contributing factors. *The major determining factors are the degree of emotionality, either overt or repressed, that is involved and the degree of local contractile tension.*

SHEN IN THE HOSPITAL

SHEN procedures have application in practically every unit in the hospital, from the cardiac unit to the maternity ward.

CANCER UNIT
SHEN is not a specific against cancer but can be extremely helpful in many ways.

The cancer patient who is facing death almost always carries a number of repressed emotions: grief, fear, negative confidence, perhaps guilt. Tensions required to contain these emotions impact on every organ in the body. A simple assessment of the cancer patient's emotional state with attention to emotions being denied will let you devise a treatment plan.

Chemotherapy Some interesting results have been noted with hospitalized cancer patient who is undergoing IV chemotherapy. With several patients whose white blood count had dropped quite low, Rearward Flows at the HT^3 region followed by HT-C, resulted in a marked increase of white cells.

Social Work Social workers find SHEN quite helpful for the family members as well.

Imagery Imagery work with cancer and other patients can be supported and enhanced by the use of Shen. The process varies from the usual one.

Specific Shen work at the cancer (or other disease) site frequently bring spontaneous images. If they come, these are prime images for the patient to work with. (Typically, successive Shen sessions with a recovering patient will bring images that are lighter in tone and with a color shift away from reds and blacks towards blues and greens.)

At any point the patient can creatively visualize these images changing towards more desirable ones. It is important that if further Shen at the site brings new and different images that the old ones be discarded and the new ones used in the imaging process. Do not dwell on the old images or on their meanings. **Returning to old images will be counterproductive.** If the imaging process works to heal, we can assume that working with older images would reverse the healing process.

CARDIAC UNIT
Some studies report that as many as 60% of elderly cardiac patients suffered a grief-filled incident within six months prior to their heart attack and that expression of that grief was denied for one reason or another. It is not difficult to see how contractile tensions to suppress grief would affect the physical heart. The tension would exacerbate any reduction in blood supply due to accumulation of plaque in the arteries. Releasing the tension and the grief can only be beneficial. (Don't neglect work at the Kath, the elderly patient losing a mate often suffers from an identity crisis.)

INTENSIVE CARE UNIT
Often the IC patient is caught in mortal fear. This is due to psychogenic shock (See Protocol page 131). In addition much can be done to increase body temperature, and to stimulate organ function.

Since the patient is often in pain and/or immobilized, work with the hands under the body should be avoided except, perhaps, at the extreme sides and then with caution. Be sure the hands rest lightly on the body. **Use caution when placing hand under body.**

PRE-SURGERY PATIENTS

SHEN is extremely helpful in reducing or eliminating complicating fear - the fear of the operation. Transverse flows at Kath, Solar Plexus, and at the trauma site are most productive. Start with the flows at the trauma site as this is likely to cause sleep, thus allowing deeper relaxation during remaining SHEN.

1. Flows through the injured or affected part from several directions followed by flow in normal direction
2. Flows at the Solar Plexus
3. Flows at the Root are often very effective. Transverse Flows if you can't get your hands underneath.
4. Flows at the Kath.
5. Finish with Peripheral Flows.

Shen also assists in reducing swelling. (See front of this chapter.)

POST SURGERY

Expectations: Shen is immeasurably helpful in promoting rest and relaxation, partly by easing pain. Swelling is routinely reduced following Shen and comfort and rest are enhanced. The reduction of swelling could be expected to accelerate healing possibly due to increase of blood and lymph circulation.

Protocol Similar to Pre-Surgery
1. Flows through the site of the operation are good but do not apply any pressure, (it is best to keep hands just above the body surface).
2. A Root to Crown flow is good if it is not uncomfortable for them.
3. Finish with peripheral flows.

LACK OF APPETITE FOLLOWING SURGERY

Shen treatments 24 to 36 hours following surgery can assist in regaining normal appetite and bowel movement. Quite dramatic shifts in appetite and BM's have been noted.

Protocol Flows through digestive organs and colon are appropriate. Also, do Frontal flows and diagonal flows from front of the body through the digestive organs.

1. Flow through Pancreas. Place RH on anterior torso at the right side of the SPH line, LH at the center of Kath.
2. Flow through the liver/gall bladder. LH at Kath, RHat left side of the SPH line. Both flows affect duodenum.
3. Flows through ascending and descending colon. Place one hand above the other, with the colon in between. Be sure the direction of flow is appropriate for the frontward or rearward line chosen.

SHEN TREATMENT PROTOCOL   **PSYCHOGENIC SHOCK & SOME COMA**
(Emotional shock and/or the emotional component of physical shock.)

Etiology Psychogenic shock is severe emotional shock with severe physical consequences. The region around the groin contracts in the face of extreme physical or mortal fear. The contraction probably affects the caudal ganglia - at the lower junction of the left and right sides of the sympathetic and parasympathetic nervous system.

Procedure
1. Relaxation flows along both sides you may want to do this in segments.
2. Transverse at Root <R>
3. Do a long Root flow. This may take several minutes and, when successful, may result in a sudden threshing of arms and legs accompanied by moans of fear. This will not last long.
4. Triple frontward at Solar Plexus SP^3
5. Triple frontward at Kath K^3
6. Root to Kath R-K
7. Root to Solar Plexus R-SP
8. Root to Crown R-C

SHEN TREATMENT PROTOCOL   **FRACTURES, SWOLLEN OR SPRAINED JOINTS**

Shen can reduce pain and swelling and can relieve tension around joints to a surprising degree. With nearly healed injuries, a Shen session may cause tremors in the affected part as small muscles relax.

1. Flows from every angle through the joint or break
2. Finish with a flow in the normal direction
3. Transverse flows at the side of the swelling that is towards the heart can be helpful.

SHEN TREATMENT PROTOCOL   **ARTHRITIS**

Shen will not end arthritis but will reduce the pain, often considerably and for increasingly extended periods.

1. Complete Peripheral flows
2. Do flows through affected joints, from every angle and follow with
3. A flow through the joint in the normal direction of body flow
4. Back to front flows at the Solar Plexus are useful
5. Finish with peripheral flows.

SHEN TREATMENT PROTOCOL   **BURSITIS**

SHEN has been very helpful with bursitis. Flows from every direction through the affected joint followed by normal arm or leg flows. I know several people who no longer have bursitis since receiving a few SHEN sessions, myself included.)

SHEN TREATMENT PROTOCOL   **KIDNEY STONES**

Considerable help can be given the sufferer of renal colic. The pain can be reduced a good amount and relaxing the region may help the passage of the stone.

Fear The person suffering from a stone is frequently afraid. Flows at the Root and at the Solar Plexus can help this.

Nausea This is often present. This can be helped by Peripheral flows at the Solar Plexus, Pubic region and by triple frontwards at the Solar Plexus.

Local Tension/Pain at the site of the stone. Diagonal flows through the region can reduce the pain a noticeable amount.

Protocol
It is best to have the patient's upper body slightly elevated, lying on their side with the pain side up.
1. Relaxation flows along both sides from the Solar Plexus to the Pubic.
2. Triple frontward at the Solar Plexus SP^3
3. Right hand on pain side of torso at the Kath/Solar Plexus line, left hand at the Pubic center. This can reduce the pain and does appear to relax the duct. You will need to stay there until the stone passes or the pain will build again.

SHEN TREATMENT PROTOCOL   **GALLSTONES**

It is possible to cause the passage of gallstones with SHEN. The patient should sit, propped up and relaxed, head resting on a support. The right hand should be on the patient's right side at the Solar Pelxus/Heart line. The left hand at the Kath center. Have the right hand quite a ways around on the back. The angle of this flow is in the direction of the bile duct.

SHEN TREATMENT PROTOCOL   **ACHES AND PAINS OF THE AGED**

Do peripherals and Root to Crown. If pains are on front have them lie on back - if back pain, have them lie on stomach.

Shen tends to dissolve minor aches. A few sessions usually reduce low level pain and keep it lowered for an extended period.

SHEN TREATMENT PROTOCOL   **MUSCLE TENSION HEADACHES**

Transverse Flows at the Throat and Mouth along with HT^3, and T^3.

SHEN TREATMENT PROTOCOL   **SINUS HEADACHES**

Sometimes drainage can be improved with Transverse Flows at the eyes and nose.

PREGNANCY AND BIRTHING

Third Trimester Shen can relieve much of the pain and discomfort of stretched tissue around and especially below the baby. Have the mother-to-be lie on her back, knees raised and supported by a pillow. Diagonal flows: K_R-RP^C followed by K_L-RP^C. Babies love SHEN, do a K^3 flow right through the baby. Spinal and Peripheral flows are good to do also.

During Labor Flows across the body through the pubic region <RP>, <P>, <PK>, ease labor pain and discomfort greatly. These flows seem to help cervical dilation.

SHEN TREATMENT PROTOCOL **VERTIGO TINNITUS**
(Also for **some hydrocephalus**.)

Etiology It is presumed that excessive fluid is in the inner ear and needs to be released. The intent is to relax the spinal column segment by segment from the bottom up, approaching the greatest tension from its farthest reaches. There is no need to go farther down than the heart.

Procedure First do relaxation flows along each side and then the head loop. (Note that the patient may notice changes in, or additional, tinnitus during this part of the procedure.)

1. Complete Peripherals
2. H^3
3. HT^3
4. <T>
5. T^3
6. Mouth (TF)
7. <Occiput>
8. <Temples>
9. <Back of Head>
10. KSP^3
11. PK^3
12. K^3
13. R-K
14. R-C

SHEN TREATMENT PROTOCOL **JET LAG**

1. Complete Peripherals
2. R-K^3
3. R-SP
4. R-H
5. R-T
6. R-C
7. Feet

PROTOCOLS FOR EMOTIONALLY ROOTED DISORDERS

The protocols that follow are general outlines of the core procedures and will need to be adjusted for the individual patient. Doubtless you will need to adjust the protocols as you proceed from session to session. Number of sessions needed can vary greatly. (The protocol for chronic low back pain is in the next chapter, on page 144)

Remember, in all cases, the patient with any of these ailments may very well have some current pain or emotional problem that is adding a layer of armor to the deeper problem. Observe the patient's breath, body posture and tensional patterns. Then begin the procedure with something that addresses those tensions. After the person begins to relax deeply, you can begin the procedures outlined here.

SHEN TREATMENT PROTOCOL   IRRITABLE BOWEL SYNDROME

Etiology
Guilt, shame, fear, impotency and anxiety are the usual precursors. Repression of these emotions through constriction of their somatic affect suppresses peristalsis and normal bowel function.

Treatment Since there is no biological cause for this disorder, course of treatment is usually short. Usually one or two Shen treatments are enough, the second session 48 hours after the first, if possible.

Protocol
1.   Relaxing flows should include sides of torso bridging the Kath.
2.   Triple rearward at Kath/Solar Plexus line KSP^3
3.   Triple rearward at Pubic/Kath PK^3
4.   Triple frontward at Kath K^3
5.   Triple frontward at Pubic P^3
6.   Triple frontward at Solar Plexus SP^3
7.   Side Flows at K_L-K^L, K_R-K^R, SP_L-SP^L, SP_R-SP^R, KSP^R-KSP_R, KSP^L-KSP_L
8.   Root to Kath R-K
9.   Root to Pubic R-P
10   Root to Crown R-C

Post Session
Usually there is a great deal of rumbling in the gut. The patient may attach shame or guilt (which is being elevated and released by the treatment) to the rumbles and express considerable mortification. Explain that the sounds and movement are quite normal, to be expected and are definite signs that the treatment is helping.

Next twenty-four hours Bowel action is likely to increase and then stabilize. This should be mentioned so as not to cause undue distress. (The patient is likely to report an improved sense of well-being that begins during this period.) **Note:** There may be a brief period of mild toxemia as old decayed fecal matter is loosened and expelled.

Etiology

A great many **Common and Classic Migraines** appear to generate at the rearward line between the Heart and the Throat (HT). This is the site of the baroreceptors on the aortic arch that control general blood volume, the origin of the carotid arteries and the aortic loop of the vagus nerve. As the migraine proceeds it may produce tension at the occiput and shoulders. (Migraine may also be preceded by tension headache.)

With migraines that respond, some kind of deep grief is the precursor, often from childhood, often involving an incident of deep sadness that includes a threat to security and sense of self. (A child grieving over parental divorce, for example, also loses personal identity, which is closely interlocked with the parents.)

Etiology

Acephalgia and Abdominal Migraine (Migraine without head pain)
and **Childhood Cyclical Vomiting** These appear to begin at the Solar Plexus/Heart line and involve fear in addition to grief. There is often a history of childhood carsickness, cyclical vomiting or biliousness. Considerable fear seems to have been evident in early childhood.

Etiology

Cluster Headache Experience is limited with cluster but it appears to stem from constrictions at the rearward line between the Heart and Solar Plexus (SPH). (A substrate of anger and fear has been clearly evident with the few I have seen.)

Treatment

Best performed during attacks but may be performed prior. It is best if they do not take analgesic medication (taken to lower pain) if they are willing to do so. (And if their meds are PRN). If they are on Prophylactic meds (taken regularly to prevent pain) they should continue to take them. Unless, of course, their doctor fully agrees to withholding the meds.

Treatment During Attack

Two or three treatments during attacks are advisable. Occasionally, one is all that is necessary, if it is conclusive. It can be considered conclusive if (1) deep sleep with REM occurs during flows at the appropriate rearward line, (2) headache ends during treatment and (3) grief loaded memory occurs that reveals some previously hidden information within 24 hours following treatment. When all three occur, the episodes may have ended. However, tell patient another migraine may occur and that you will do another session then.

Treatment Between Attacks

Usual course is three treatments just prior to attacks, additional treatments may be necessary if the patient does not relax fully during the procedures. Very deep relaxation should be seen during one of the treatments, specifically while flows are being done at the principal rearward line. Sleep, REM and snoring are not uncommon. NOTE: memory of precipitating event may not occur, even if series ends.

(Continued on next page)

Procedure (Same for treatments during or before attacks.)

1. Relaxation flows along both sides of the torso, bridging heart region
    NOTE: Flows around the head will likely increase headache pain.

2. Once relaxation starts, do rearward flows;
    (a) HT^3 for Common and Classic
    (b) (SPH^3 for Cluster, Acephalgia, Cyclical Vomiting.)
    NOTE If the headache is unilateral, start on the side opposite
    the pain, i.e. with a Rt. Side Common Migraine: HT^L, HT^C then HT^R.

3. Triple frontward flows on both sides of rearward line:
    (a) T^3 and H^3 for Common or Classic.
    (b) (H^3 and SP^3 for Cluster, Acephalgia, Cyclical Vomiting.)
    Do these long enough to get a full flow.

4. Repeat Step 2 if deep sleep did not occur.

5. Do the other rearward flow, either above or below heart (triple).

6. If treatment is during attack do:
    A. Transverse flow across occiput and follow with:
    B. Transverse across shoulders.

7. If migraine ends during session do K^3

8. Do R-K, then extend to:

9   R-H and finish with:

10 R-C.

Migraines with Nausea/Vomiting

To relieve the nausea or vomiting and to release the anger/fear underneath you will need to do these flows:

SPH^3
KSP^3
SP^3

Menstrual Migraine

Session for menstrual migraine should be scheduled for the day of the attack, usually the first day of menses. You will want to include:

PK^3
KSP^3
K^3
P^3

Secondary Gain

Note: Migraines often become imbedded in the dynamics of unsatisfactory personal relationships. It may be the only time the sufferer gets cared for, or time to him or herself. If this is the case, he/she may do some psychosocial gyrations to offset the missing secondary gains, may raise tension headache to migraine status to justify stronger medication, or may fail to show up for their Shen treatments.

Sometimes migraines become mixed with muscle or sinus headaches. See page 132 for treatment suggestions.

PREMENSTRUAL & MENSTRUAL DISTRESS
DYSMENORRHEA EXCESSIVE BLEEDING

Etiology
Typical profile reveals poor self image. (This has nothing to do with their image as seen by others or with their effectiveness in day-to-day functioning.) The roots of this syndrome are in early childhood. (Children are often made to feel impotent or are taught to feel shame when there is no valid reason.) Involuntary constriction of the somatic affect of shame and impotency takes place in the Kath region, the site of the ovaries. These early tensions remain in place but have minor effect until the ovaries begin to function. Situations that increase the feeling of impotency exacerbate the condition.

Treatment
Very effective when there is no contributing organic cause.

Premenstrual or Menstrual Distress Plan three sessions, one on each of three successive months, on the worst day of the symptoms. (Often two sessions are enough.)

Excessive Bleeding, Dysmenorrhea Plan for three sessions, one on each of three successive months, on the first day of menses.

Menstrual Migraine For additional information, see the Migraine Protocol, Page 135-136.

Procedure Patient should be supine, knees raised on pillow for comfort.
1. Relaxation flows should include both sides of torso bridging kath.
2. Transverse at the Pubic/Kath line <PK>
3. Triple frontward at Kath K^3
4. Triple rearward at Kath/Solar Plexus line KSP^3
5. Triple frontward at Kath K^3
6. Triple frontward at Pubic P^3
7. Root to Pubic R-P
8. Root to Kath R-K
9. Root to Heart R-H
10 Root to Crown R-C

Note: If the patient begins to cry at any point a brief frontward flow at Heart will accelerate the process. Then resume the procedure. It may be necessary to reassure the patient that it is all right to cry or to release other emotions since not all women have accepted the freedom to be emotional that is assumed to be their natural right. (It is best to do this by saying "Good", "Yes" "OK" when the tears start, rather than start an intellectual discussion on the benefits of tears.)

Post Treatment
Patient should understand that if effective, there will be some alteration in flow, ovarian chemistry and associated emotions.

Etiology

The psychological picture of the anorectic usually includes: (1) unresolved parental conflicts from childhood, and/or (2) unrealistic fears of gaining weight (3) fear of food.

The emotions involved, anger and fear, both include somatic affects that present at the **Solar Plexus** and **Epigastric** regions. Repression of these somatic affects adversely effects function of the liver, gall bladder, pancreas, spleen and stomach, thus directly converting the emotions of anger and fear into anorexia and other eating disorders.

Treatment

Intended to release the constrictions around the digestive organs. This stimulates the organs towards normal functioning. Release of the somatic affect may promote the emergence of the associated emotions of fear and anger and, possibly, related memory.

Protocol:

1. Relaxation flows along both sides of torso, bridging Solar Plexus.
2. Triple rearward at Kath/Solar Plexus line KSP^3
3. Triple rearward at Solar Plexus/Heart line SPH^3
4. Triple frontward at Solar Plexus SP^3
5. Extra frontward flows at sides of Solar Plexus $SP_R\text{-}SP^R$, $SP_L\text{-}SP^L$.
6. Diagonals, front to back: $SPH^R\text{-}KSP_L$, $SPH^L\text{-}KSP_R$.
7. $KSP^R\text{-}KSP_R$, $KSP^L\text{-}KSP_L$
8. If deep sleep/REM occurs repeat frontward triples at Solar Plexus SP^3
9. KSP^3
10. Triple frontward at Kath K^3
11. Root to Kath R-K
12. Root to Solar Plexus R-SP
13. Root to Crown R-C

Post Treatment

If the treatment produced physiological responses, ie. reflexing, REM, the patient should be advised that they may go through a short period of emotional turmoil possibly including brief, mild stomach upset. There may also be a night or two of nightmarish dreams. They need to understand that these are signs of progress.

CHAPTER 18

SHEN AND CHRONIC PAIN

Because of its unique ability to access emotional causes of pain, SHEN work has uncovered several previously clouded aspects in the etiology of chronic pain. The result is a unique perspective on pain that has led to several interesting treatment developments. One of these is a specific intervention for migraine that frequently ends the migraine series in mid-attack. This and other SHEN interventions are currently in use as primary modalities at several chronic pain centers.

SHEN has a high success rate with a number of types of physical pain refractory to other methods of pain control, and is effective with all psychogenic pain manifestations. This psychogenic factor frequently plays a large part in the total pain syndrome of primarily physical or biologically derived pain. SHEN treatments eliminate the psychogenic portion of chronic pain, the part not continuously regenerated by an ongoing biological process.

PHYSIOLOGICAL RESPONSES TO PAIN

The typical reaction to pain of either physical or emotional origin is one of automatic avoidance. Avoidance reaction is through physical withdrawal by constricting or rigidifying the region of pain. These constrictions, which embrace non-contiguous muscle groups and non-muscle tissue alike, pervade and stress the entire region of pain. Since the causes of these avoidance reactions are often long term, the constrictions tend to become permanent. By the time the originating cause ends, the process often becomes embedded in the body as it loses its ability to relax the localized pockets of constriction. *What was useful has become harmful.*

Pain is at the interface of the physical and the emotional. Since the avoidance/constriction patterns are the same for both, these reactions become inextricably tangled when they occur at common sites. This is a vital factor in chronic pain. It is through this common denominator of locality that long term emotional pain combines with the pain of injury or disease, converting into chronic pain that persists long after its visible cause has ended.

MAJOR PAIN COMPONENTS IN CHRONIC PAIN SYNDROME

The existence of several active elements or components in the phenomena of chronic pain has been repeatedly confirmed by the results obtained from SHEN Therapy treatments. These are the *biological, protective and emotional* components. While any of these may stand by themselves, more than one is necessary for chronic pain syndrome to exist. The relative percentage of each will determine the course of the pain, its duration and its treatment protocol.

BIOLOGICAL COMPONENTS

Biological pain results from nerve and tissue damage, and is a byproduct of pathogenesis or biogenesis. The biological component ends when the tissue regeneration ends. While the biological component is not always the original element in the chronic pain syndrome, it is usually the one which exacerbates the condition into visibility. While the ongoing biological process continues to generate pain, SHEN will usually provide temporary relief, but the pain will not be eliminated.

PROTECTIVE COMPONENTS

This element is caused by involuntary guarding reactions to the core pain from a blow or break. When the initial physical pain occurs, the common reaction is to withdraw from it by constricting the region around the pain site to prevent it from hurting. Immobilization is useful because it assists the damaged tissue in moving as little as possible in relation to adjacent tissue. This immobilzation, called the *splinting reflex,* assists the healing process in the same way a cast assists a broken limb. This component is involuntary and may not end when the biological pain ceases.

Figure 92   Development of Simple Chronic Pain

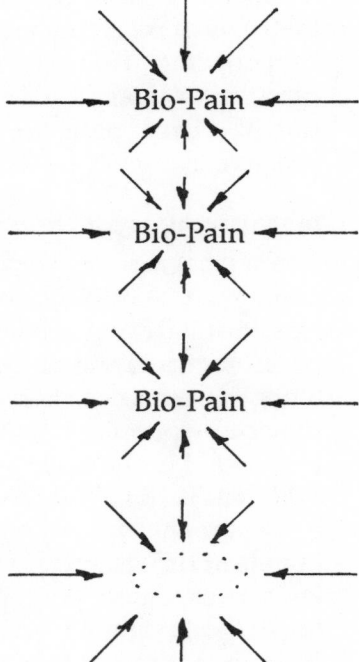

1.   An injury occurs and biological pain begins.

2.   Tissue is constricted around the pain site to immobilize and contain the pain. The constriction is involuntary and not subject to conscious control. The patient is unaware of the constricting effort.

3.   In time the constrictions become automatic.

4.   The tissue at the pain site heals, but the constriction remains and is now the source of pain.

This is the simplest form of Chronic Pain, as most Chronic Syndromes include emotional complications.

EMOTIONAL COMPONENTS

INJURY RELATED EMOTIONAL COMPLICATIONS

There are two injury or accident related emotional elements in Chronic Pain. One is caused by emotions being experienced as the injury occurs and the second by emotions generated as a result of the injury.

PRE-INJURY FEAR

Frequently fear reaction to an impending accident is an important complication. The impending accident is perceived with fear and results in a tightening or constriction of the entire body. This tensing places the body in a detrimental posture when the accident occurs. Not only does the tissue suffer more damage then it would if flexible during the accident, but there is evidence to suggest that the tensions become locked in the body tissue by the shock of the accident itself. Therefore, the constriction does not end when the tissue heals and the biological pain component ends.

Patient "A", member of special police squad, injured when he fell from a ladder during training. The incident was particularly fearful because he fell backwards, striking the small of his back on a blunt projection. Although there was no evidence of physical damage, the pain had not abated in five months. Currently on sick leave. Questioning showed he did not fit the profile of the chronic pain patient with poor self image. To the contrary, he glowed when talking about his job and presented a strong, somewhat macho, attitude. He was deeply concerned about being transferred to a lesser (less risky, less interesting) job.

He was advised that we could not tell until after the treatment whether it would be beneficial, but that if it helped, the pain could probably be eliminated in two or three treatments. He did not appear to be overly excited but was game to try. Inside of ten minutes his back had noticeably relaxed and softened and he was in deep sleep. When he woke thirty minutes after the treatment, the pain was entirely gone, replaced by delighted amazement. The following day minor pain appeared around his shoulders, apparently as a result of releasing the previous tension in his lower back. A second Shen treatment brought relief to his shoulders and regular workouts in physical therapy brought no new pain beyond the expected sensation of muscles being brought back into use. His pain never returned.

POST-INJURY FEAR

A similar reaction is prompted by the fear of discovering how much damage really exists. In this case the constricting may be partially conscious, but just as hard to overcome as the patient is unaware that he or she has translated the fear into the physiological constrictions. The physiological reactions, the pain remaining after the biological cause ceases and the response to SHEN treatments are all similar to the previous example.

NON-INJURY RELATED EMOTIONAL COMPLICATIONS

A great many studies have shown that psychological or emotional factors are involved in many chronic pain syndromes. A high percentage of chronic low back pain patients, for example, have personality profiles that include *poor self image*. It is very difficult to either treat or understand the etiology of this back pain on the basis of poor self image. It is much easier to follow the process by which poor self image converts into lower back pain when it is considered from a site-related emotional perspective rather than from psychological or personality perspectives.

There is a very precise site-related relationship between the emotions involved in poor self image and in chronic low back pain. The emotions that present in poor self image are feelings of, or lack of, confidence and guilt. The bodily sensations with both of these emotions appear at, or just below, the navel. (Terms such as *gutless* in reference to the person who displays no confidence and *I was gutted* illustrate the location of the sensations.) Vertebrae L4 /L5/S1, the ones most commonly involved with chronic low back pain, are in the navel region.

The somatic feeling sensations that present at the navel/L4/L5/S1 region are removed from somatic awareness by constricting that area. This tends to become endless because, if ever relaxed, the unpleasant somatic affects will reappear. The result is that the musculature around the spine loses its resiliency and becomes vulnerable. When this already stressed region is subjected to further stress through strain or injury, the stress effects combine and any physical damage will be greater than would be expected for the strain or injury alone. The pain associated with the injury will be greater than expected and will last longer, becoming chronic in many cases.

Since no internal mechanisms are readily available to end them, this combined tissue stressing results in significant chronic pain. (It is not necessary for a physical injury to occur in emotionally stressed regions in order to produce chronic pain. It is well known that pain, such as the chronic low back syndrome, can occur independent of injury to the region.)

EMERGENCE OF MEMORY

In releasing the constraints surrounding the somatic sensations in this type of chronic pain, SHEN treatments often trigger the release of the long forgotten emotion that produced them. In turn, this often releases related memory or episodes of abreaction.

Patient "B", Plumber. Strained and injured his back (L4/L5/S1) during a routine job operation. The disc between the vertebrae was badly swollen. During his first SHEN treatment, which focused on that region, REM was observed twice and later he reported two memory flashes. The first involved a fight with his father and the second was the memory of proposing to his wife while thinking he would be rejected. He was so startled by these spontaneous memories that he wondered if he was losing his mind. (He was assured that he was not.) Both incidents were heavy with emotions of guilt and lack of confidence. Pain abated following the treatment but, because of the severely swollen disc, did not end.

Figure 93 Development of Complex Chronic Pain
The Fusion of Emotional Pain and Biological Pain

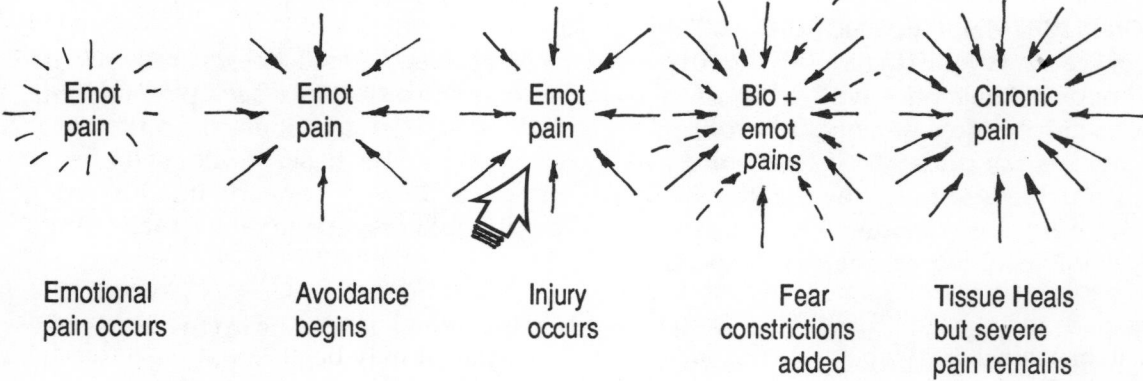

Emotional	Avoidance	Injury	Fear	Tissue Heals
pain occurs	begins	occurs	constrictions	but severe
			added	pain remains

PSYCHOGENIC PAIN

Psychogenic pain is pain in which the contributing cause has been forgotten and the emotional component covered with time. Both the originating situation and the specific emotion involved are hidden from view, with only the psychogenic pain remaining to indicate the presence of an unresolved emotional trauma. These cases are interesting for the SHEN therapist because they often present the most unique and colorful histories. In many cases the treatment releases "memory" of events that could not have happened. While these cannot be explained as ordinary memory, the metaphor is usually quite clear.

Patient "C", Salesman, Age 40. Severe low back pain without organic cause. CAT scan and other tests negative. Pain continuous since childhood, flared under stress. Had increased to present level three months prior. Ate pain pills like candy, with about the same effect. His body relaxed noticeably at one point during the SHEN Treatment. His first words after the treatment were "I'm not going to say it doesn't hurt because you didn't do anything". After a few minutes he added, "I remembered being stabbed in the back, but nothing like that ever happened to me". He never did admit that the pain was gone, but he stopped taking his pain pills. Six months later, when asked how his pain was, he snapped "What pain?" and walked away.

Frequently the patient's metaphorical dreams and fantasies are useful in determining the treatment protocol.

Patient "D" Suffered a minor injury to his wrist. Shortly afterwards he began to have severe pain centered in a small area in the forearm near the elbow. Tunnel syndrome was suspected and the nerve canal was opened with no change in pain. After enduring several months of pain and consulting with nine different specialists (one of whom re-performed the operation without result), he was desperate. During questioning by the SHEN Therapist he revealed that he had had a strange daydream episode while dozing in which he felt that his arm had been severed. He was questioned as to how much of the arm was missing. "I felt flat from here down" he said, indicating his shoulder.

The procedure to be used was not discussed with the patient. He reclined and an EMG unit was connected directly across the pain site. The session began with the therapist placing his hands across the region of pain. Later, as the patient relaxed and drifted into a light sleep state, the therapist performed a SHEN procedure at the "amputated" shoulder. During the course of treatment the EMG indications dropped 95%. When the patient awoke he said, with obvious amazement, "When you put your hands on my shoulder a jolt of energy shot from my shoulder into my head and the pain stopped. I've got to admit that it's back a little bit now, but when you put your hands on my shoulder it all went away." Subsequent treatments reduced the pain even more.

SHEN TREATMENT PROTOCOL UNREMITTING PSYCHOGENIC PAIN FROM A STRONG BLOW

Sometimes pain from a strong blow will not leave even after extensive SHEN. A procedure that is practically guaranteed to help (where there is no biological cause for the pain to be there): Do a flow through the injured area placing your hands so you do a flow in *exactly the reverse direction to the force of the blow*. It may be necessary to extend your LH a foot or two off the body. (I can't explain why, but it works.)

Figure 94
To reverse the
force of a blow

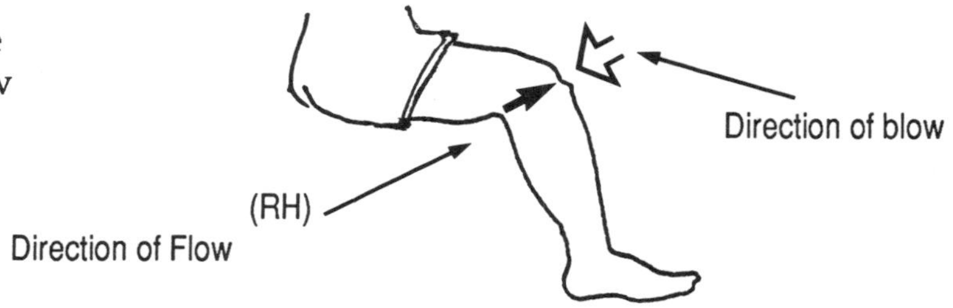

Direction of blow

(RH)

Direction of Flow

Etiology Poor self image is high on the profile of the LBS patient. This self image generates emotions of shame and impotency (usually beginning in early childhood) with somatic affects presenting at L4/L5/S1. Repression of these somatic affects stresses the region, causing minor pain in its own right and setting the stage for severe strain upon relatively minor exertion. Treatment effectiveness will be determined by the degree of this psychogenic factor in the total pain.

Treatment Several are usually necessary. The effects are cumulative. Treatment is usually best with patient prone. Support stomach and torso to relieve lumbar strain. If procedure is done with patient supine, support knees with pillow.

Procedure
1. Do Peripheral flows along each side, from P to SP.
2. Follow this with transverse at Kath <K>
3. Spinal flows, first with hands about three inches above and below K.
4. Then increase this spinal flow in segments till R-C is reached.
5. Follow with transverse at the Pubic/Kath line <PK>
6. And transverse at the Kath/Solar Plexus line <KSP>
7. And transverse at the Kath <K>
8. Rearward triples at KSP^3
9. Rearward triples at PK^3
9. Then triple frontward flows at the Kath K^3
10. Root to Kath R-K
11. Root to Crown R-C. *(You may wish to do SHEN Flows at the throat.)*

Note: If a major flexion occurs during the sequence, remain there for two or three minutes. Follow this with a frontward flow at K and then resume.

Post Treatment Inquire about memories, images, emotions. These may be painful and sometimes tearing occurs. Remember crying is thought "unmanly" by many men. Reassure patient that the release of these emotions is normal.

Expectations Degree of effectiveness will depend upon the degree of physical damage present. (1) Where there is no physical damage the LBS may end in one session (2)those with damage take longer but biological healing will accelerate when the psychogenic factor has been released.

Caution Release of the core pain and lumbar tension will provide an increased range of motion which should be explored gently as the tissue in the region may not regain full strength for several weeks.

Next Day Frequently when the core, or central pain is released, secondary pain(s) occur around the periphery of the body, particularly the legs and shoulders. These result from the re-posturing of the body caused by the relaxation of the lumbar muscles. Reassure the patient that this is a good sign, showing that things are getting back to normal. Shen treatments at the secondary pain sites are appropriate. Caution the patient against over stretching or over exercising.

DETERMINING THE DEGREE OF PSYCHOGENISITY

In chronic pain, just as with other suspected psychosomatic syndromes, there is always a question of just how much is "Psycho" and how much is "Somatic". Determining this is quite simple. When the pain was/is entirely somatic, one of two things will happen when SHEN is performed. (1.) There will be NO effect. (2.) The pain will end and not return. This is rare, however, as there is almost always some psychosomatic portion.

EXPECTATIONS WITH THE PATIENT WITH CURRENT SOMATIC PAIN
1. Fully healed: Rapid results. Pain can leave in one session but more likely will be followed by pain in other parts of the body. This occurs because tension is like a spider web, break one part and the connections at the other ends knot up in bunches. This is what the muscles do when the central tension ends.
2. In process of healing: Pain relieved for several hours at a time, better sleep.
3. Not healing: Little effect, any gains are rapidly lost.

EXPECTATIONS WITH THE PATIENT WITH PSYCHOSOMATIC PAIN
1. Totally psychosomatic. Can end rapidly but it will release repressed emotion if it does. Sometimes bewildering to the patient - who can't believe the pain they have carried for so long could evaporate so fast.

2. Psychosomatic with an injury on top of the emotional pain. There will be a consistent lessening until a shift in the results occur. The shift occurs when the emotions suddenly start to be released after a few session without any, only effects on the pain.
   a. The range of emotions is likely to shift from day to day.
   b. Deeper issues, not directly related to the original complaint begin to emerge.
   c. The physical symptoms decrease in intensity as the emotional ones increase.
   d. Pain seems to move outward from the central point to new areas.

All this is quite normal and requires that the therapist be on his or her toes and stay with what is happening now, not on where the patient was yesterday. This change of events must be brought to the attention of the psychotherapist in charge. The big problem, however, is with the patient. The patient had no idea those emotions, memories and problems were under the surface and may be quite startled by their surfacing. If the idea of emotions or of losing control is frightening, the patient may think that he/she is, "Losing my mind". Improperly handled, the patient will lock down on the emotions, causing more pain and the creation of new ones. But, this well may be a rich time in the patient's life, one ripe with change for the better. It will depend on the patient's psychiatrists, counselers and psychotherapists.

SAFETY OF SHEN

SHEN is entirely non-invasive and may be used directly at the pain site without discomfort to the patient. SHEN is effective with a great number of pain disorders, especially those with a psychogenic component. SHEN combines well with other treatment modalities and is augmented and supported by Bio-feedback and other relaxation techniques.

PATIENT MANAGEMENT AND CONCERNS

There may be brief emotional episodes following release of very long term pain. These should be encouraged in a thoughtful manner. Patients in the depression that sometimes follows severe, permanent physical trauma may find that their suppressed fears and sadnesses are elevated into consciousness and may temporarily feel that life has no meaning. The usual cautions and counseling will apply. It is better to have this occur while under treatment instead of later, as appropriate precautions can be taken to safeguard the patient.

PHYSICAL THERAPY

Ideally, these approaches should be altered when the protective or emotional pain components cease, as release of the tensions will alter the relative musculature configuration. (You may wish to refer to Chapter 14 COMBINING THERAPIES page 115, for information on merging SHEN with massage and with imagery techniques.)

PATIENT RESPONSE

SHEN is quite well received, often being requested by patients who have observed its benefits with other patients.

SECTION V

APPENDIX A   **CASE HISTORY** _____ _149_

APPENDIX B   **THE SHEN NOTATION SYSTEM** _____ _163_

BIBLIOGRAPHY _____ _165_

INDEX _____ _167_

Appendix A

CASE HISTORY

These verbatim case notes are presented as an example of the results of using Shen Therapy with emotionally rooted disorders. It illustrates many of the types of experiences that can occur during Shen sessions, the emergence of hidden memory and the rapid changes in psychological functioning that can occur as a result.

"S" Age 46 Migraines since age 28

Takes ergotamine regularly (inhaler) - feels they bring on the migraines as well as stop them. Was told ergotamine withdrawal takes 12 to 21 days to get past the migraines caused by withdrawal. Migraines usually on right side. Usually begin with creeping pain up back of neck, then hatband, then migrainous behind eye.

History

First migraine was just before her period at age 28. For one or two years they seemed to be of 48 hours duration occurring on Thursdays, but that was probably because here periods were regular. Her doctor took her off birth control pills and she was without migraine for two months. She was given a prescription for Ergomar, which she took for four years (till 1974 or 75, about age 34). At that time an incident occurred which was overwhelming and she had a severe migraine (and vomited for the first time). Switched to Caffergot PB suppositories. Gradually began increasing use until she was taking them daily. This continued until 1979 when she was taken off Caffergot because she began to be worried about addiction.

About one year later (1980) got an Ergotamine inhaler. Used it only occasionally until July 25, 82, when she went back to Boston for her 25th class reunion and forgot her inhaler. Her period started the day of the reunion - had a horrible migraine that lasted two days. (But had a good time at the party.)

From 1980 until six or eight months ago was taking Ergotamine daily at onset. However for the last six or eight months has taken Ergotamine every night in anticipation of having a headache the next day. Takes it whether she has early signs or not.

The first migraine that lasted four or five days was last October (85) following her attending an "Erotic/Exotic Ball". She said "I must have been traumatized, but I enjoyed it." (Seemed puzzled by why she would have been "traumatized" since she clearly wanted to go and had enjoyed the evening.) This was about the time she began taking Ergotamine in anticipation of attacks.

During the last four years, the longest time without ergotamine (one time only) was about 2-1/2 days but otherwise 48 hours was maximum. Lately, the maximum time between migraines is 24 hours.

Results of using Ergotamine inhaler.
1. Effects vary but usually whatever kind of headache, (migraine, tension or mixed) she takes Ergotamine for, the pain will either go away within an hour or the pain will dissipate until it becomes nagging, finally ending 5 or 6 hours later.
2. When a migraine starts she takes Ergotamine, goes home and lies down. The migraine may go away in 4 or 5 hours, but not always.
3. Sometimes if she has a "nagging" headache and takes Ergotamine the headache gets worse and then goes away however, over the last three or 4 months they haven't gone away as they used to.

Last ergotamine at 5AM Sunday (Today).

1st Session   Sunday afternoon July 27, 1986

Migraine in first phase, some aura at right eye. Slightly nauseous feeling, tension pain back of neck and around eyes. No migrainous pain yet.

Session lasted about 30 minutes. Did standard migraine protocol. Heart/throat line from left to right. At right side sobbing began and continued through Solar Plexus/Heart line and Heart line. Sobbing ended.

S: "It's not sadness like it was before, there's joy in it too because I can see where I've been. (Quiet for a while) "Just thinking - when I get deep inside - the truth is there".

"The first feeling I had was when your hands were at my breast. What does this mean - can I trust? What I've learned tells me not to trust. I'm naive, felt like my mother was saying 'How could you be so stupid.' The feelings faded-" (Actually, therapist's hands were not on her breasts but above them.)

"Then thinking about my dad - an incident when I was four - I asked my mother why I was an only child. She said, *"There were two reasons, because we can't afford any more and daddy didn't want children, he didn't want to take responsibility, but he loves you"*. Felt like (pause, deep sigh) may have been the first horror I ever felt - real bad news."

"When your hands were here (indicated just below her navel) I was thinking about being pregnant with my sons - it was very painful, lonely, at times I felt abandoned. "Then when your hands were back at my heart I was thinking of a friend I saw say this morning - how she is going through a sacred time of her life (Friend is dying). Feeling close to God - feeling how far I've moved - yearning - pain- the agony/ecstasy around that - the beauty of it."

"Thoughts about my relationship (with J., her lover) - I sent him away - When I'm with him I lose myself. Pain and sadness - frustration - confusion and a lot of love. How deeply I love and how much it hurts."

"Recently I had connected the memory of being told about my father not loving me with (the time) when I became reluctant to kiss him good night. (But) This time (I remembered it) I physically felt it - like a draining out - a terror. Like so many times I've gotten bad news - swallowed it and went on. (Pause) My father killed himself when I was 18."

Note: It is typical to have the actual emotion of an event that was previously remembered but without emotion, surface during a SHEN session.

2nd Session Monday 8:30 AM 28 July 1986

Interim:
Woke with incipient signs of migraine headache. Did autogenic handwarming exercises which helped. She arrived with vague traces of the onset aura.

Session:
Did Heart/Throat line and solar Plexus/Heart line followed by heart line. Much sobbing following session.

S: "Tried to go back (to remember) to where I was in the first session. Felt like they didn't want me after they got me. Flashed to my husband - when he got me *he* didn't want me. Scenes of our apartment - felt like a tomb. My stomach felt like it did all those times I vomited with migraine - like suffocating - like I'd died."

"Still feeling like I want to throw up - like something coming down over me - depression. Used to get up on Saturday mornings and stare out the kitchen window - like I had died - like no hope, it could never change."

(Decided to continue the session. Worked at Solar Plexus) Got a very good flow at the Solar Plexus, breath changed.

R: *"What happened?"*

S: "It just went peaceful (pause) "I saw flowers outside the window."

R: *"The kitchen window?"*

S: "Yes" (Brief tears - sobbing) "I didn't know it had it in me then".

Note: The re-remembering of an event with images of an opposite nature to those previously recalled indicates the beginning of change in the person's life - in this case the emergence of hope.

S: "Its no wonder I freak out when somebody wants to marry me". "It's amazing - it's all in my body - I feel all the pain of the emotions."

Note: The times that she had recalled these events prior to recollection during the SHEN session were emotionless, without affect.

(Continued with Shen flows at the head to reduce the hatband pain)

S: "I realize I've got a choice whether to take the Ergotamine or not."

R: "You can chose between taking the Ergotamine or looking at the flowers." (In reference to the recall of flowers outside her window.)

3rd Session Monday July 28, 86 5:00 pm, just after work

Interim:
S: "Had a late lunch - began to feel nauseous - took aspirin which doesn't work. Felt immensely better after lunch. My forehead feels like it is full of tears, just like it does before crying."

Session:
Did Heart/Throat line, Mouth and then Throat. At throat she became agitated, left hand began picking viciously at bumps in her slacks, feet began twisting. - dry sobs began. Did flow at forehead much more sobbing. Then flow at Solar Plexus.

S: " It's making my head hurt".

(Later after more desolate sobbing) R: *"what are you feeling"*

S: "Like being frozen - being bound with ropes."

Later the crying sounded quite young - right leg began futile kicking.

R: *How old do you feel?"*

S: "4 - 5- 34, I don't know"

R: *"4"* (because it sounded like a four year old.) Sobbing deepened and intensified. Began doing flows at the Kath. Sobbing went on a long time - deep wailing sound - gradually faded out.

Susan sat up, scratched her head, made a face and said "Not any fun, Richard" then laughed. "My forehead was awfully painful for while - not as much now - I don't feel quite as nauseated - part of it is I think I can't feel - a blanket of nausea, of despair over everything."

R: *"What was going on?"*

S: "Lots of things. Thinking about my sense of helplessness as a child - If I hurt or if things would happen my mother wouldn't take up for me. She would say *"What did you do"* (or) *"You've got to take care of yourself"*. When you asked how old I was all I could see was a photograph of me in a Halloween costume at age 3 or 4 - thought how adorable that child was - and it hurt so much. I never felt like I was that adorable little child."

"Earlier (in the session) felt I was going back into that apartment (The one she lived in when married) - didn't want to - getting drunk and having fights - my husband hitting me and I would say I was sorry. Still carrying that now - always needing reassurance - never enough. When I was 5 or 6 a big girl beat me up mother said *"You've got to take care of yourself.'"*

"Sunday afternoon my parents would go to bed to take a nap and leave the radio on to the baseball game - I wandered around - abandoned - hating the sound of the game. And I still do that now when I hear a baseball game."

"It was the same nauseated feeling I had this morning (during the Shen session) about my apartment (with former husband) - and that's the feeling I get when I think about getting married now. (And) the feeling doesn't have anything to do with the present. The other feeling is of getting drunk and being sick."

Note: At this point she began making mental connections between the emotional feelings and the physical feelings.

4th Session Tuesday July 29, 1986 7:45AM (48 hours since Ergotamine)

Interim - Overnight:
S: "I Went home - felt real bad across my head, felt better by the time I got home - swam - felt ok, small pain in my stomach. Ate dinner at 8PM. Decided to visit J (her lover that she sent away a week ago) was feeling the 'migrainey feeling' on my left side. (Not the usual side) Could feel stuff about my father, sons, (ex)husband - but felt positive. We made love."

"He wanted me to stay the night - was angry when I didn't want to so I agreed to stay - realized I always succumbed when others were angry. Later I could feel a migraine starting to come on, told J. that I'm working on these migraines and I can't stay. He agreed and I realized that he wasn't angry after all, I just thought he was. So I went home.

I went to bed with the beginnings of a migraine - was certain that I would have a severe headache in the morning (still didn't take the ergotamine). Dreamt about my (ex)husband - not upset about being with him at all - didn't have the 'Oh my God I've gotten trapped' feeling" (Which she always has during her frequent dreams about her ex husband).

Note: Her feelings about her ex-husband are beginning to change.

Session: Worked at the Solar Plexus/Heart line - at left side a sudden deepening in breath and some eye movement. On the left side of the Heart line - breath still deeper. At the left side of the Solar Plexus line sobbing began, moved to the center of the Solar Plexus and the sobbing went on a very long time. Sounded quite young - like crib age.

Afterwards she sat up, grimaced and said, "Oh God, can I see the line (meaning the connection between events in her life) I can see exactly why I chose J. I kept going back to the little girl with the pumpkin - so cute and so alone. Allowed myself to get into my rage at my father - he never looked at me - never took care of me - I couldn't depend on him. Daddy always had a problem - not knowing who he was - I remember how my uncle was different - couldn't depend on him (father). Then I had thoughts of my father's suicide when I was 18 - I had to drop out of school and stay home to take care of mother."

"It was the same with my husband, couldn't depend on him - would get phone calls from his office saying they were sending him home - I remember the doctor saying he was referring him to a psychiatrist. (Husband was manic depressive with psychosis). I couldn't get angry at him and now I've chosen a man who doesn't have a job. Well, actually it's different; he had a job until three years ago when he went on a sabbatical to find out who he was - mid life crisis, I guess. (But) he had enough money put away to support himself. Now he's looking for a job because the money is about to run out. I don't want to take care of anybody else. There is still some nausea and my head still hurts. I still want to throw up."

5th session Tuesday July 29, 1986 5:30pm

Interim - During the day:
S: "Felt alright during lunch, got worse about an hour later. I'm sick to my stomach, pain has gone up over the right side of my head mostly around head in a band. This (headache) is (a migraine of) about a 7 on a 1 to 10 scale."

First part of Session:
Right side of Heart Throat line: REM and shoulder twitch. Right side of Solar Plexus Heart line: REM, breath change, mouth and nose twitched. Right side of Solar Plexus: Noticeable breath shift - slower fuller. Center of Solar Plexus: Hips moved, frown, mouth and hands moved. At Right shoulder, twitched two or three times. Throat light snoring then very relaxed breathing. Transverse flow at the shoulders: mouth opened wide and distorted. Transverse at mouth , mouth opened wider, light crying began. Hands began fighting the pad under her, crying got louder and continued. Raised her knees and thrashed around a bit. Flow at Heart and at Kath evoked continued crying which finally subsided.

R: *"How do you feel?"*

S: "Head is clearer, migraine feeling still there but it has shifted, not as severe".

Second part of session:
Asked her to lie on stomach. Did side flows then section of the spine from about the Kath to the Heart. Then transverse flows at Solar Plexus followed by a flow through Solar Plexus back to front. She relaxed quite a bit.

R: *"Little better?"*

S: "Yes there is still some tension.

R: *"Some of it is muscle tension that will take time to go away - lot of new stuff this time?"*

S: "Yeah, strange - feeling grateful to be peaceful and I was almost dreaming.

R: *"You were, I could see it - Rapid Eye Movement and snoring".*

S: "(laugh) And then I could feel the energy moving through my body I could **feel**, - felt good-grateful to feel peaceful - I didn't want to really get into anything because it would hurt. Then you put your hands on my shoulders and it was like going right back to when I was about 6 and my molars were pulled. I had to have them extracted and they put me in the hospital to do it. And I had had my tonsils out a year or two before and I remembered the ether and it was just awful and I remember being wheeled down to the operating room and I was yelling by the time they got me down there and then they were going to put that ether - and then I felt my mouth open - and you remember when my mouth was open? - I hadn't put it together but then I remembered they put a thing in my mouth and tied my hands down and -.

R: *"Well that explains everything that I saw."*

S: "It was like I was feeling all that - and then when I was bringing my legs up it was like when I was trying to fight that - they were real angry with me. My mother wouldn't do anything - of course she couldn't but I wanted her to stop them - she wouldn't - I remember screaming and the horror of having them tie me down and put that thing in my mouth."

R: *"I wondered yesterday when you spoke about the feeling of being tied down, what was behind the feeling".*

S: "Yah, I could feel that, it's funny because I remembered that (the incident) but without the emotions - the rage - the helplessness - tied down. You know I remember that - the horror, just the horror that somebody would actually do that to me!"

Note: This time the recall included the previously suppressed affect.

S: "And then I went up (her thoughts moved on in time) to when I was in the hospital to have my first child and my husband - my husband had gotten terrible during the pregnancy - staying out until all hours - getting drunk - finally about a week before I went into the hospital I had undeniable truth that he had been fooling around with women. The previous times he had denied it but this time it was undeniable and this time he admitted it, said he felt so awful - he had all these women's cards in his pocket - and I went into the hospital and had the baby and that wasn't so bad - I didn't mind having the baby. The hardest part was lying in the hospital knowing what was going on with my husband. And I couldn't do anything about it - they were playing soap operas (on the hospital TV) and it was like my life going on (in the soap operas) and I couldn't get them to turn it off."

"Then the real funny part was that I went back (thoughts went back in time) to when - all of a sudden - I could feel myself - it was almost as if I didn't have arms and legs but I did, I was a person, and I was very little, and I was walking around my house looking for my mother and I couldn't find her."

(She explained) "Well, they told me that when I was about 6 months old she had a nervous breakdown and they had to put her in the hospital."

And I felt myself walking around saying "Where's Mommy, where's Mommy?" and then there was this awful feeling of where is she, where is she?. And I could sense my grandmother's presence and then I walked to the door of the bedroom and it was like there was a body dead on the bed. And I don't know what that was about - it was a heavy, horrifying feeling and I have no

154

idea - I have never had that imagery or those feelings. But I was very, very small and I could feel myself almost like a little 'schmoo' - remember them? - The shape is what I felt like. And that was it - that was awful".

R: *"Well, sounds like we're getting pretty deep doesn't it?"*

S: "Yah".

R: *"Lot of unraveling".*

S: "I notice that one of the things I do when I get tense is opening my mouth like that."

She left intending to try not to take the medicine and to exercise some. Susan, "Feels more migrainey then I did last night."

I Reminded her that she can look at the flowers.

6th session Wednesday Morning 8:00 AM July 30, 1986

(Susan phoned before coming, "I'm dying and it's not fast enough".)

Interim:
S: "Fell asleep watching TV - woke - felt fine went to bed - No real bad dreams, but something about children. (In the dream) I was late to work, had clothes in the drier, was just very late and my mother was there and I decided to let her help me - I was just very late. (I had) anxiety because of that but it wasn't a bad dream. I woke at 3 felt horrible, woke at 5 couldn't go back to sleep. I ate a small breakfast."

Headache on right side, "Like a rod rammed through" from right side occiput to right arch of eye socket by nose, nasal drip right side. (Face very gray), brought a pail to vomit into.

Session (First part):
Progressive relaxation during flows at Solar Plexus/Heart line, and Heart/Throat line. Flow at center of Solar Plexus produced gurgles in intestine and marked change in breath pattern during flow at right side of Solar Plexus, breath deepened - turned head to right side and relaxed into pillow. Color returned, more gurgles, solar plexus region softened. Another flow at the Solar Plexus induced a very large gurgle. Seemed to be asleep. (25 minutes elapsed since start of session.)

S: "Stomach still hurts - not as bad - feel peaceful. The birds (that she heard outside the window) were bringing back memories of the '40's - picket fences, roses, children playing in the back yards. Seeing myself when I was real little - I was alone a lot - just feeling all the places I was in - I would feel myself on Grandmother's lap. I was feeling a sense of confidence that I had way back then.

Richard *"So how old were you?"*

S: "4, 5, 6, maybe a little younger. Remembered times when the kids started being mean - don't remember what mother said but I got scared - I think she told me I just had to accept it or (possibly) that it didn't happen. Such a sense of freedom - of totality - of being on the earth - believing in myself. No restraints - being who I was - just playing.

R: *"Why don't you stay with that feeling?"*

S: "For the rest of my life?"

R: *"Yes"*

S: "Do you remember what the gardens were like in the 40's? - green grass - flowers - white fences - summer mornings - back in the East, days when it wasn't real hot?"

R: *"Yes - what is the feeling around your eye?"*

S: "Sharp pain" (indicated from right temple to arch of right eye and nose and pain from occiput to arch of eye and nose).

Session (Second part)
Did flow from left eye to right temple. Tears started, increased, became intense. Changed flow: from left eye to right occiput and then did flows at Throat, Solar Plexus, Kath and again at Solar Plexus. Crying continued throughout.

R: *"Are you feeling sorry for yourself?"*

S: "I just hurt".

R: *"Where?"*

S: "Inside" more tears - crying stopped, and she sat up.

R: *"Feel a little different?"*

S: "Yeah, still don't feel good - I feel like my whole body is kind of buzzing. I started thinking about that feeling. Feeling the loss - then - that memory about my mother telling me about my father. She was standing in the front yard and I was standing there looking up at her - and I started feeling that it was - like my body was shaking - feeling like standing there having her tell me that. Could feel the little girl there with her arms plastered down at her sides, standing on her feet, like cement had been poured over her - and the rage at the hurt - having that taken away from her. (Sense of confidence she had been feeling). That was the sense of can't trust, that was the feeling that - that was the point at which I stopped trusting the universe. Feeling like I'm not supposed to be here - it's not right to be here - like it's not mine. And that beautiful child - I just have a sense of what a beautiful child I was.

R: *"Could you say 'Beautiful Me?'"*

S: (Laugh) "Yah, beautiful me - I know it's going to take a while for that to sink in."

R: *"Not as long as you think."*

S: (Some crying) I was absolutely totally trusting - I was just standing there listening to her - oh my God - I couldn't trust. I never felt this before - it was like I was in that body - I just felt dark - like all the sunlight in the garden went away. Don't know if it did."

(I discussed how tunnel vision occurs when one is upset by a sudden emotional shock.)

"How do you get past that - now that I've recognized that how do I change?"

R: *"After what you've just gone through, (in these sessions) why do you think your not past it? You've broken the tensions in your body that were holding those emotions in. The tensions in the body were what put the pain in your body."*

S: "That was the other thing - I was angry that I should have to have all this pain - angry." "It's amazing that you can hold a memory - I could see the scene - but I never felt it. It was like I disassociated.

R: *"It is like the emotional quotient of the memory has to come up, until that happens you can't ever get rid of it."*

S: "That's why I feel that I don't fit or don't belong. It didn't feel like just that day in the front yard. It felt like I had made some horrendous mistake - can't explain it - it felt so universal."

R: *"How does your body feel?"*

S: "It doesn't bother me, feel much more relaxed, pain in my head is not as severe, more like a real bad tension, not as pervasive. Still want to throw up." I invited her to do so, she left and did. Returned and said, "First time I've been sick to my stomach since 1980" (When she left her husband). Well I'm much better now, this morning I didn't think I could put one foot in front of the other."

7th session 5:30PM Wednesday Afternoon July 30, 1986

Interim:
Arrived somewhat gray. "Still sick at lunch, was going to go home but one of the men gave me a job that just had to get out. Realized that the feeling I got this morning was that I didn't belong on the planet. Just thinking about it (the memories) - when I do I feel nauseated, depressed.

R: *"Are those emotions the ones you feel when you have the migraines?"*

S: "The thing - the thought - that goes through my body - is how that affected me. And I feel angry, awareness of the beauty of the totality of the human being. The sense of the rightness of being on the planet. Got a sense of my mother being the messenger between my father and myself. I was always giving her presents, I was four, I was always telling my friends what a grouch my mother was.

R: *"What are you feeling now?"*

S: "Nausea, tightness in this muscle (pointed to muscle at right occiput) It starts here and goes over the top of my head to my eye. Doesn't feel as bad as this morning. My nose keeps running on my right side."

First part of Session:
Reclined on stomach. Did transverse flows starting at about the Solar Plexus and moving up in bands to the throat. She relaxed quite a bit. Then did flows from front to back at Kath/Solar Plexus line, Solar Plexus/Heart line, Heart/Throat line and neck. Myoclonic jerks at all. Lots of 'heat' in my hand. Flows up right side produced big jerk and shudder. Flows across occiput and across scalp - much stinging heat in my hand.

R: *"How do you feel?"*

S: "Peaceful"

R: *"Head?"*

S: "Still hurts but it is peaceful. It is like a lot of movies going on in my head. Was getting pictures of another family. At times it felt like I was the mother and father and other times the child - (we were) a unit. They were very concerned about the child. I tuned into the sacredness of having this child - Very serious concern. Then it felt like I was the child and I was being taken away against my will - like something had happened - don't know - remember what - something dark."

They were very light beings - very bright - like lighted from within. Funny, I could see my two parents standing there, like something was happening - some trouble - but they are not worried about themselves - worried about protecting the child - I was scared. I can feel hands taking me away - pulling me away. Feels like they took me away and swung me around and killed me by hitting my head on something.

Then I was seeing my two sons - thinking 'Gee all of this seems to be about men."

R: *"How's your body?"*

S: "Still nauseous head about the same. (Her face is much clearer and good color, seems very peaceful.) Some of the memories are so heavy they make me nauseous - its so depressing."

Second part of session:
Reclined on back. Intestinal gurgles when flow was done at Kath/Solar Plexus line. At Kath, much heat in my hand, Solar Plexus again - big gurgle and shudder."

S: "Something I forgot from before - (earlier this session) when you had your hand on my shoulder it felt like being held down with my head under water. Now it is almost as if the pain is there to block the thinking.

When you moved your hand down to the Kath - I remembered being 4 to 6 years old, would get in the closet with my cousin and we would look at each other. Once we got caught, I had brought a little box to see how we peed. My aunt opened the door and saw us - she caught my cousin - he got spanked - I ran and hid in a box - I can't remember what I felt - I felt bad about getting caught, felt remorse, shame. Later we taught each other to masturbate felt shame over that."

R: *"That explains why you got so upset and had a terrible migraine after going to the 'Erotic/Exotic Ball'."*

S: "This is pretty intense stuff - It's amazing how I've been through so much therapy but it only touched the surface of it, but I was detached from it - but that's the thing, we detach from our feelings."

8th Session Tuesday Morning 8:00 AM July 31, 1986

Interim:
"Went to bed late. Little bit of nausea and migrainous headache feeling. Dreams: "(I was) In a house with my inlaws - having a bad time relating to them. Boring talk, not interested in it - I stood up and found I was wearing only a silky nightshirt with nothing under it. Grandmother said 'Do you not wear underwear Susan? I thought 'Oh, my god', was angry and left. Saw myself in a mirror - looked like a young man, was startled, image in the mirror had short hair and no makeup. Then I remembered that when I put on a dress and makeup I look like a woman and I like the way I look."

(Then) I Walked into a room full of young people, the TV was loud, told them 'You've got to turn that down' - felt guilty - realized , gosh I'm angry - I can't be Mrs. Nice any more.

Then I was sitting in a circle of women who were passing plates with a little cookie on each plate - said to myself 'I can't stand this' - felt very out of place.

Then I was in a truck going uphill following another truck, I was afraid the truck (in front) was going to fall back on me - the trucks were full of old furniture - we ended up at a place that looked like a huge garage sale. There was this old used furniture spread all around - trying to get rid of it - above all it was furniture from back in the '40's. We approached a counter and realized we were going to see our old furniture."

I Woke at 3AM, ate, still had head symptoms, not as nauseous. Woke at 5AM felt lousy couldn't got to sleep again. Felt better after eating this AM." Color good, eyes tired.

Session:
Flows at Solar Plexus/Heart line, Kath/Solar Plexus line, Solar Plexus and Throat lines. No crying or particular body reactions.

S: "I (intentionally) kept going back to the memories I had yesterday, (but I) couldn't get into it. When your hand was at my throat I felt that I wanted to scream at my father to come alive - he was so remote - feeling a lot of anger about that.

Then I was thinking about how I fall into old patterns when I'm around my parents. (For example) when I'm with them I sit around and drink Mahattans which is what my stepfather likes to do - (But) I never make a statement of who I am - my kids make statements about who they are but I've never done that. (Then I was) Thinking about my son - that I can't hang around his life style - never claiming my own identity. (Pause) - Like its alright to be separate from my parents and its alright to be separate from my kids. (Pause) There is something really different about the way I'm feeling about that."

9th Session Friday Morning 8:00AM August 1, 86

Phone call: "Richard I think its about done - I feel much better".

(On arriving) Good color, did not seem to be too tired.

S: "(I have) A little bit of stuff in back of neck a little in the forehead and some nausea - I did eat a good breakfast".

Interim:
S: "Last night it (the migraine) was leaving - a half hour ok than a half hour bad, a half hour on and a half hour off. Last night at the party I ate sushi and shrimp which felt real good on my stomach. Felt pretty much all right - in and out. By the time I went to sleep I felt it was pretty much under control. Woke 2 or 3 times but without that awful pain. I don't remember any dreams last night".

"I realize that I've never really established my identity with my mother. Two memories come back to me about that. When my mother was here on a visit we were with a friend of mine and later my friend said *"You disappear around your mother"*. Visited my psychiatrist and took my mother along, later my psychiatrist said *"You really let your mother take over, you defer to her"*. Seems like it comes from trying to keep her happy - because it's not worth it when she isn't."

Session:
Flow at the Kath/Solar Plexus line - intestinal gurgle, flow from mouth to occiput - slow tears which developed into intense crying followed by her stretching out and beating the bed with one hand in rage. (Real tears with the sobbing for the first time.)

She sat up quickly - eyes bright, almost a sparkle and said, "I think that was it, Richard (pause) it was incredible - It's just fascinating (smiled) That was Mildred - that's my mother."

Note: This is the first time she has used her Mother's name.

S: "I could feel my arms wanting to break out - (there was) no incident - it was pervading - she had me bound up in a shroud - once the arms could go I was feeling the rage - she would not let me be happy - first she had to make me unhappy - before she let me be happy - she made me unhappy before she let me be happy, she made me unhappy before she let me be happy! Feeling how she was always the one who - (voice trailed off) then she was not my mother any more just a force.

Where it got to - I don't know which came first - I just smashed her - she was a little brown thing and I just smashed it and smashed it and smashed it until it became little and I became big."

I remembered the fairy tale - the Snow Queen - and then (the one about) Hansel and Gretel - I smashed the Snow Queen and then I broke the cage (Hansel's and Gretel's) and smashed the witch - I kept smashing and kept getting bigger.

She (her mother) was the one that told me about Daddy (This was the first time she referred to him as 'Daddy', it was always 'My Father') - She was the one at the hospital when they tied me down - she was the one orchestrating this pain in my life."

R: *"How do you feel?"*

S: "Excited" - I could feel her hand coming down on me there (indicated the muscle in back of her neck) where I get the muscle tension - I didn't feel guilty about killing her."

R: *"How does your body feel?"*

S: A little funny stuff on the top of my head and tightness from crying - my stomach is not upset at all, my stomach feels fine. I wonder if my Mother has a headache this morning. I feel like I have been trapped in the niceties of the world."

She left, smiling.

Tenth Session Saturday Morning 9:30AM August 2, 1986

Stomach shaky, panicky, neck tight, tension, light headed.

S. This morning I realized that the image of me as a gargoyle killing my mother was because I'm angry. I've had this feeling of wanting to kill, to tear something apart before.

Session:
Flows at the Kath/Solar Plexus line and at the Solar Plexus evoked crying and kicking. While doing flow at the Kath I told her to relax her arms and legs, she let go and the tension drained. (Much heat in my hand at the Kath.)

At this point the phone rang and the answering machine picked up the call (the answering machine was by the bed where we were working). It was from her mother, the machine amplified the call and S. began sobbing, almost whimpering.

R: *"If you won't talk to your mother like a grown woman I guess you'll have to stay being a little girl."*

After a few minutes, more tears. Lots of heat at Solar Plexus and Heart. Tears came fully just before session ended.

S: You know, she has the capacity to reduce me to nothing - just with the tone of her voice. In the beginning (of the session) I was just letting the images come in - they were real vicious - I should paint them - I often have scenes in my head - weird gargoyle-like creatures - mostly red. I started thinking about my artwork. (A brief discussion of art techniques followed.)

"When I heard my mother's voice - that tone - I feel like I could throw up when I hear her - belitteling - and it hurts - and all the anger and strength I had yesterday left. When you said what you did I started imagining myself talking over her, talking past her.

R: *"How do you feel"?*

S: "Real tight, my head feels a little tight".

R: *"What can you do about it?"*

S: Relax.

R: *"Why don't you talk to your mother? You only have one choice, you know, you can either be angry at your mother or angry at yourself."*

Monday AM August 4, 1986

(Phone Call) S: "I called my mother on Saturday, she wasn't home so I didn't get to tell her that I was angry at her. But it was real funny - I got to listen to my stepfather tell me about how he was angry at her and all the details of that."

"Sunday I felt fine until 5PM when I was slightly migrainey - I ate late, still headachy - was afraid that it would be bad this morning - I woke at three and did my autogenic handwarming - I'm feeling great this morning - had a dream about my son.

Tuesday AM August 5, 1986

S: "Woke at 4AM with a feeling of nausea. Woke again at 5AM with increased nausea and realized that there were emotional feelings of panic as well. Realized what I was feeling panicked about.

"J. is planning to go on a trip without me. I can't go because I can't afford it and I have to work. I've been upset and didn't quite know why - then it hit me - once when I took my (former) husband to the airport to send him off on a trip - just as he was getting on the plane he told me "I'm meeting a woman on the plane and we're going on this trip together. I was stunned and couldn't react - I got out to my car and got hysterical."

"Then (this morning) I began to cry - I was in the shower and just cried and cried - when I got out of the shower my nausea (and panic) were gone."

161

Note: This is an excellent example of the conversion of an emotion (panic) into a physical disorder (nausea). The physical tension necessary to contain the feeling of panic (at the Solar Plexus) was so strong that it produced nausea in the stomach and duodenum.

Tuesday PM August 5, 1986

S: "I'm feeling great".

POSTSCRIPT

Later, in February of 1987, she had three migraines, each immediately following being involved in an activity about which she had extreme misgivings. As soon as she came to a clear decision to stop the activity, the migraines ceased.

APPENDIX B

DEFINITIONS, LOCATIONS AND NOTATIONS

DEFINITIONS

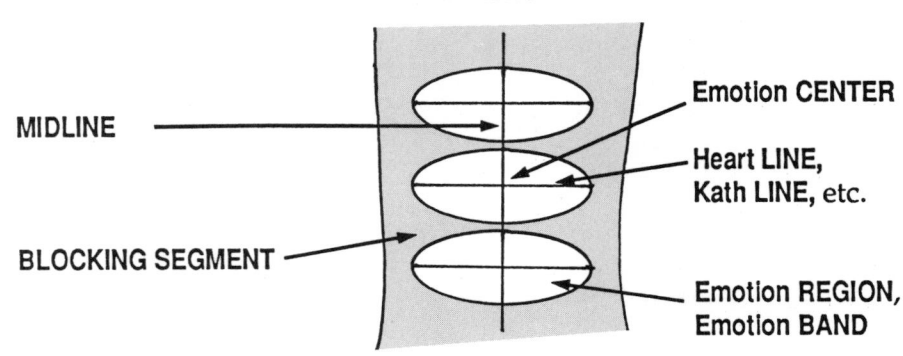

MIDLINE

Emotion CENTER

Heart LINE,
Kath LINE, etc.

BLOCKING SEGMENT

Emotion REGION,
Emotion BAND

LOCATIONS

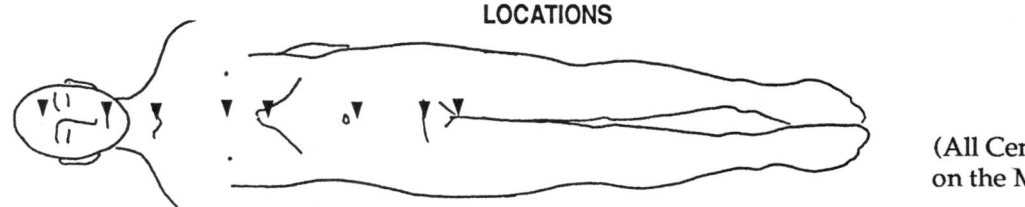

(All Centers are
on the Midline.)

Forehead	An inch above the eyebrows.
Mouth	Upper jaw line.
Throat	At the notch where the sternomastoids join the sternum.
Heart	Midway between the Throat Center and the xophoid process.
Solar Plexus	At the xophoid process (the cartilage below the sternum).
Kath	An inch below the navel, on a line with the iliac crests.
Pubic	At the upper edge of the pubic bone.
Root	At the junction of the legs/lower buttocks crease.

NOTATIONS FOR ANATOMICAL LOCATIONS

Star Point	*	12 to 24 inches above head, at edge of the field
Crown	C	(Top of Head)
Forehead	F	(Just above eyebrows)
Mouth	M	(Upper Jaw Line)
Throat	T	(Notch where the sternomastoids join the sternum)
	HT	(between Heart & Throat)
Heart	H	(Center of chest)
	SPH	(between Solar Plexus & Heart)
Solar Plexus	SP	(At the xophoid process - cartilage below sternum)
	KSP	(between Kath & Solar Plexus)
Kath	K	(Inch below navel, on line between the iliac crests)
	PK	(between Pubic & Kath)
Pubic	P	(Upper edge of pubic bone)
	RP	(between Root & Pubic)
Root	R	(Junction of legs/lower buttocks crease)

DEFINING THE EMOTION REGIONS AND BLOCKING SEGMENTS

Cross section of the
body at the KATH
viewed from the Feet

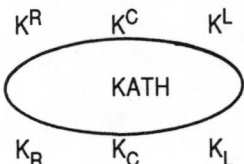

Except for the Forehead and Mouth, all Emotion Regions and Blocking Segments have three hand positions on the front and three on the back. Use $^{\text{Superscript R,C or L}}$ for the upper positions and $_{\text{Subscript R,C or L}}$ for the lower positions.

SHORTHAND NOTATIONS FOR THE TRIPLE FLOWS

To record doing all three flows in a Emotion Region or Blocking Segment, follow the letter with a $^{\text{superscript3}}$. For example: for three flows at the Heart use H^3, three at the KSP Segment use KSP^3.

SEQUENCE OF SHORTHAND NOTATIONS

The written sequence of the notations indicates the direction of the flow as the location written first is always the location of the **SENDING HAND**. Therefore the notation R-K indicates a flow from the Root to the Kath. Remember that the sending hand is **always** on a site that **receives** (where the normal flow of energy is inward) and the receiving hand is **always** on a site where the normal movement of energy is outward.

SHORTHAND NOTATIONS FOR THE ROOT FLOWS

These always begin with an R and follow with a center as in R-P, R-H.

SHORTHAND NOTATIONS FOR THE CROWN FLOWS

In RP-C for example, the Right Hand is at RP, the Left Hand at the Crown.

SHORTHAND NOTATIONS FOR EXPANDED ROOT AND CROWN FLOWS

Just put the $^{\text{superscript 3}}$ following the notation you would ordinarily use for the Root or Crown Flows: $R-K^3$, $R-H^3$ or SPH^3-C, HT^3-C, etc.

SHORTHAND NOTATIONS FOR THE TRANSVERSE FLOWS

Transverse Flows can be either direction (except across the shoulders whre the flow should follow the person's arm flow). Examples: <R> <RP> <P> <PK> <K> <KSP> <SP> <SPH>.

SHORTHAND NOTATIONS FOR THE FRONTAL FLOWS

Note the position of your Right Hand, then a dash, then the position of your Left Hand. RP^L-H^L, RP^L-H^R, KSP^R-T^R, KSP^R-T^L.

SHORTHAND NOTES FOR SIDE FLOWS

The two locations look the same, except for the subscript and superscripts: Frontwards; K_L-K^L, H_R-H^R, and Rearwards: KSP^R-KSP_R, HT^L-HT_L.

BIBLIOGRAPHY

Almy, T. P, L. E. Hinkle, Jr., B. Berle, and F. Kern, Jr. Alterations in colonic function in man under stress-III. Experimental production of sigmoid spasm in patients with spastic constipation. *Gastroenterology* 1949,53 821-833.

Alexander, F. *Psychosomatic Medicine*. New York: Norton, 1950 *Psychosomatic Specificity*. Chicago: University of Chicago Press 1968.

Bartrop, R. W., Lazarus L., Luckhurst E., Kiloh, L. G., Penny R., Depressed lymphocyte function after bereavement. *The Lancet*. 1977, 1 pp 834-836.

Engel, B. T. Stimulus-response and individual response specificity. *Archives of General Psychiatry*, 1960,2 305-313.

Engel, B. T., & Bickford, A. F. Response specificity: Stimulus-response and individual-response specificity in essential hypertensives. *Archives of General Psychiatry*, 1961,5, 478-489.

Fromm-Reichmann, F. *Psychoanal. Review*, 1937, 14,1.

Grace, W. J, & Graham, D. T. Relationship of specific attitudes and emotions to certain bodily diseases. *Psychosomatic Medicine*, 1952, 14, 243-251.

Reid, R.L., & Yen, S.S.C. Premenstrual syndrome. *American Journal of Obstetrics and Gynecology*. 1981, 139 pp.85-104.

Schwartz, G. E. Psychosomatic disorders and feedback: A psychobiological model of disregulation. In J. D. Maser & M. E. P. Selisman (Eds.) *Psychopathology: Experimental models*. San Fransisco: W. H. Freeman, 1977.

Sternbach, R. A. Autonomic responsivity and the concept of sets. In N. S. Greenfield & W. C. Lewis (Eds.), *Psychoanalysis and current biological thought*. Madison: University of Wisconsin Press, 1965.

Sternbach, R. A. *Principles of psychophysiology*. New York: Academic Press, 1966.

INDEX

Note: CASE HISTORY Listings and SHEN
TREATMENT PROTOCOLS can be found
on page xiv.

A

Abreaction, 13, 24
Aches and pains, 132
Affect, 6
Affect, somatic, 6, 29, 47
Anatomic locations, 92, 65
Anatomic specificity, 11
Anorexia, 138
Anxiety,
  attacks, 118
  chemical, 52
  emotional, 52
Appetite loss, 138
Arthritis, 131
Auditory hallucinations, 118

B

Back pain, 141-144, 17-19, 21
Bands,
  emotion, 68, 69
  Reichian, 69
Biochemistry,
  and emotion, 51-54, 39, 42-43
Biofield, see:
  physioemotional field
Birthing, 133
Bleeding, menstrual, 137
Blocking segments, 68, 699
Blow, effects of strong, 143
Body regions, 29, 69, 11, 12
  epigastric, 22, 23, 14, 12
  gastrointestinal, 15, 14
  heart, 24-27, 11, 12, 14
  hypochondriac, 22, 23, 14, 12
  iliac, 20, 21, 14, 11, 12
  low back, 17-19, 14, 12
  lower gastrointestinal,12,14-16
  perineum, 27, 28, 14, 12
  pubic, 20, 21, 14, 12
  umbilical, 17-21, 14, 12
Body sensations, 81
Bones, broken, 32, 131
Bowel, 134, 16
Brain action, 49-51
Brain,
  emotional, 47
  visceral, 47
Breath, 71

Breathing, 78, 109, 111
  biphasic, 111
Breathwork, 115
Broken bones, 32, 131
Bulimia, 138
Bursitis, 131

C

Cancer, 129
Capillary perfusion, 31, 32
Care, intensive, 129
Cardiac care, 129

CASE HISTORIES, see page xiv

Centers, emotion, 87,66,68,47
  compression of, 68
  field action at, 66
  interferences at, 68
  location, 66
Chemotherapy, 129
Children's night terrors, 121
Chronic low back pain,17-19,141-4
Chronic pain, 139-144
Circulation in the field,68,65,64
Client,
  concerns, 122, 146, 121
  explanations, 33, 37
  instructions, 114
Clouds, formation, 64
Colon, 134, 16
Coma, psychogenic, 131, 27
Combining other therapies with
  SHEN, 115-116
Commanding self, 47
Compression at emotion centers 68
Concerns, patient, 121, 146
Confused thought, 50
Confusion, 50
Contractility, 7, 8, 31, 33
Contraction, 9
  around painful somatic affect 8
  automatic, 7, 31, 32
  epicenter of, 10
Conversion disorders, 6, 26
Conversion, experience into
  expression, 40.
Course of treatment, 112-113
Crohn's disease, 138
Currents, rotary, 64

D

Definitions, 87, 165-166
Degree of psychogenisity, 145
Depression,
  major, 117, 121, 118
  psychotic, 119, 121
Differences, stress results,10-12
Direction of flows, 79
Disfunction,
  approaches to, 33-35
Disorders, (also see name)
  conversion, 6
  emotionally influenced, 128
  emotionally rooted, 5, 134
  psychosomatic, 6
  somatoform, 6
Dreaming, 119, 13

E

Eating disorders, 120
Ecstasy, 124
Effects,
  of efforting, 77
  of polarity, 60
  polar, field, 60
  psychogenic, 5
  psychoplastic, 5
  relaxation, 13, 59
  stress, 10-12
Emotion, (also see Emotions)
  altering brain function, 47-51
  and biochemistry, 42, 43, 52-54
  and body movement, 40
  and brain function, 47-49
  and sound, 66
  and vibration, 66
  as a field, 45, 55
  as a puzzle, 38
  bands, 68-69, 87
  centers, 66-69, 47, 87
    compression of, 68
    field action at, 66
    locating the, 66
    vibrations at, 66
  composition, 42, 43, 47-53
  controlling, 48
  effects of repressing, 29
  essence of, 39
  differences between
    biochemistry and, 51, 53
    thoughts and, 47
  direct perception of, 45, 46
    another person's, 45
    from a spiritual guru, 45

  in group meditation, 46
  in mass hysteria, 46
  on entering a room, 45
    person to person, 45
  field-like effects of, 45, 55
  in the body, 41
  influencing thoughts, 47-50
  interferences between, 68
  mental model, 47
  perceived location, 41
    of fear, 53
  regions, 87, 88, 12, 69, 14
  sites, 47, 88, 12
  somatic, 1
  stress results, 10, 42
  transmission of, 45
    another person's, 45
    from a spiritual guru, 45
    in group meditation, 46
    in mass hysteria, 46
    on entering a room, 45
    person to person, 45
Emotional brain, 47
Emotional control, 48
Emotional differences in stress
  40, 10-12
Emotional experience, 48
  location of, 12, 29
Emotional expression, 48
Emotional disorders, 117, 120
Emotional feeling, 40
Emotional regions in the body, 11
Emotional repression, 40, 29
Emotional self, 47
Emotional tension, 40
Emotionally rooted disorders, 5
Emotions, (also see Emotion)
  and language, 12
  effects of repressing, 29,23,27
  specific, 12, 11, 29
Energy,
  field, 58-60, 75
  subtle, v
Epinephrine,
  and fear 52, 53
  stimulated by drugs, 53
Evidence of a field, 57-60
Expectations, 145
Experience of emotion, 6, 40
Experimental measurements, 58-60
Explanations to patients, 33, 114
Expression of emotion, 6, 40
Eye movement, rapid, 13

F

Falling Out, 124
Feeling emotions directly,
  from a spiritual guru, 45
  from another person, 45
  in group meditation, 46
  in mass hysteria, 46
  on entering a room, 45
  person to person, 45
Fear, 9
  and epinephrine, 52-54
  and pain, 140, 141
Field,
  direction,
    arm and hand, 76
    body, 62-63
    peripheral, 62
    spinal, 62
  effects in brain, 45, 55
  measurement of, 58-60
  nature of, 58
  patterns, 61, 64-68
  polar effects, 60, 61
  polarities in, 67, 62, 63, 65
  sensations in, 57, 75
  sensing, 75
  systems, v
Fight or flight response, 52-54
Flow direction, 79
Flows (also see Field),
  arm and hand, 76, 78, 63
  body, 62, 78
  combining, 103, 104
  crossing of, 70
  crown, 94
    expanded, 99
  emotion center, 83
  emotion regions, 83,
    94-98
  frontal, 100
  frontward, 88
  head loop, 81
  increasing the, 63, 75
  magnetic, 62, 65
  merging, 79
  patterns, 61, 64, 66, 60
  peripheral, 62, 80
  rearward, 88
  reversing, effects of, 61
  root, 83
    expanded, 99
  self, 109
  sensing, 75, 57
  shorting the, 79

  shoulder/head, 90
  sides, 102
  spine, 62, 82
  transverse, 93
  triples, 88
  weather, 62, 64
Formation of clouds, 64
Fractures, 131
Frontal flows, 100
Frontward flows, 88

G

Gall stones, 132, 110
Gastroenteritis, 138
Gestalt, 116

H

Hands,
  energizing, 63, 75
  scanning, 111
  sending and receiving 80,76
Hallucinations, 118, 121
Halo, 62
Head loop, 81
Headaches,
  cluster, 135, 27
  migraine, 135, 25, 26
  muscle tension, 132
  sinus, 132
  tension, 132
Heart attacks, 129
Helices, 64, 65
Helix, 64, 65
Hidden memory, 142-3, 149-164, 11
  13, 15, 17, 19, 20,

HISTORIES, CASE, see page xiv

Hydrocephalus, 133

I

Imagery, 115, 114, 129, 149-164
Improving organ function, 128
Increasing the field, 75
Individual stressors, 3, 11-12
Instructions
  for the client, 114
  for SHEN Flows, 78, 105, 113
Intensive care, 129
Interferences between centers, 68
Interventions,
  examples: CASE HISTORIES, p.xiv
  treatments: PROTOCOLS, page xiv
Irritable bowel syndrome, 134, 16

J

Jet lag, 133

K

Kidney stones, 132
Kreiger, Dolores, v
Kriyas, 125
Kundilini crisis, 123-126

L

Language and emotions, 12
Lines, 87
Links
  emotional, 5, 6
  neural, 5
  physioemotional, 5
Locations, specific, 87, 92, 65
Low back pain, 141-144, 17-19, 21

M

Major depression, 117, 120, 118
Management considerations, 121,
  146, 14, 121
Massage, 115
Measurements, of field effects,
  58-60
Meditation,
  ecstasy 124
  pain during, 123
Memory, 15, 17, 19, 20, 11
  emergence, 142
  hidden, 143, 149-164, 13
Menstrual bleeding, 137
Menstrual distress, 137, 11
Mesmer, Franz, vi
Metaphor, 19-21, 114-115, 149-164
  use of, 143
Midline, 87, 167
Migraine, 135-36, 25, 26, 149-164
Models,
  of health
    involuntary contraction, 35
    psychosomatic, 34
  of emotion
    biochemical, 39, 42, 43, 51
    mental, 47
Mortal fear, 27

N

Nature of physioemotional field,
  58
Neural brain/body links, 5
Nightmares, 119, 121
Notations, SHEN, 165, 166

O

Organ function, improving, 128
Organic factors,
  in tension, 32

P

Pain, 127, 139
  after ecstasy, 124
  and post-injury fear, 141
  and pre-injury fear, 140
  chronic, 139, 144
    complex, 142
    simple, 140
  components, 139, 141
  during meditation, 123
  emotional components, 140, 141
  from a blow, 143
  of the aged, 132
  psychogenic, 140-145
  responses to, 139
Panacea, 127
Pathways,
  emotional, 35
  involuntary, 35
  neural, 43
  psychosomatic, 34
Patient,
  explanations, 33
  instructions, 114
  management, 122, 146
  selection for studies, 14
Patterns,
  in the field, 61, 64-66, 68
Perfusion, capillary, 31, 32
Physical disorders with
  emotional results, 128
Physical therapy, 146
Physioemotional,
  field, vi
  link, 5
  patterns in, 61, 64-66, 68
  reactions, 32
  stress results, 42
  tension, 13
Physics,
  and emotion, 39, 45-47
  laws of motion in, 61, 62, 64
Placebo, 2, 14
Planning,
  the session, 111, 114
  the treatment course, 112, 113
Polarities, 57, 60-62
Polarity Therapy, v

Practice sessions
 class,
  Day one,
   first, 80
   second, 82
   third, 83
  Day two,
   first, 91
   second, 93
   third, 94
  Day three,
   first, 101
   second, 105
  outside,
   first 85
   second, 86
   third, 95
   fourth, 96
   fifth, 97
   sixth, 98
Pregnancy, 133
Premenstrual distress,135-7,11,21

PROTOCOLS, see list, page xiv

Psychiatric disorders, 117-121
Psychogenic pain, 140-145
Psychogenic shock, 131, 27
Psychogenisity, 145
Psychosomatic
 concept, 33, 34, 6
 disorders, 6
Psychotic depression, 119, 121

R
Rapid eye movement, 13
Reactions,
 contractile, 7, 31
 emotional, 7
 rebirthing, 115
Recall of memory, 11,15,17,19, 21
Receiving hand, 80, 76
Reflex, splinting, 8
Regional stress effects, 10, 42
Regions, body, 29, 12, 11, 69
 epigastric, 22, 23, 14, 12
 gastrointestinal, 15, 14, 12
 heart, 24-27, 14, 12, 11
 hypochondriac, 22, 23, 14, 12
 iliac, 20, 21, 14, 12, 11
 low back, 17-19, 14
 lower gastrointestinal,14-16,12
 perineum, 27, 28, 14, 12
 pubic, 20, 21, 14, 12

umbilical, 17-19, 14, 20, 21,12
Regions of
 emotion, 12, 14, 69, 87, 88
 somatic affect, 12
Reich, Wilhelm, 69
Reichian bands, 69
Relaxation effects, 13, 59
REM, 13
Response,
 fight or flight, 52-54
Results of stress, 42
Review questions for
 Chapter 2, 30
 Chapter 3, 30
 Chapter 4, 36
 Chapter 5, 36
 Chapter 6, 44
 Chapter 7, 56
 Chapter 8, 72
 Chapter 9, 84
 Chapter 10, 106
 Chapter 11, 106
Rolfing, 116
Rotating currents,
 in fields, 64, 65, 67
 in weather, 64

S
Scanning, 111
Scheduling sessions, 112
Schizophrenia, 118,
Secondary pain, 141
Segments, blocking, 68, 69
Self,
 commanding, 47
 emotional, 47
 lower, 47
Sending hand, 80, 76
Sensations,
 in body, 81
 of the field, 57, 81
Session
 planning, 111, 113, 114
 scheduling, 112
SHEN,
 combining with,
  breathwork, 115
  gestalt, 116
  imagery, 115, 129
  massage, 115
  rebirthing, 115
  Rolfing, 116
 general instructions for, 78,
  105, 113

in the hospital, 129
  temperature rise during, 32,
    58-60
SHEN Notations, 165, 166
SHEN Shorthand, 165, 166
SHEN THERAPY AND
  aches, pains of the aged, 132
  alcoholism, 119,
  anorexia, 138, 22
  anxiety attacks, 118
  appetite loss, 138, 22
  arthritis, 131
  auditory hallucinations, 118,
  back pain, 141-143, 17-19, 21
  birthing, 133
  breathwork, 115
  broken bones, 32, 131
  bulimia, 138, 22
  bursitis, 131
  cardiac care, 129
  chemotherapy, 129
  children's night terrors, 121
  chronic low back pain, 141-144
    17-19, 21
  chronic pain, 139, 142-144
  coma, psychogenic, 131, 27
  course of treatment, 113
  Crohn's disease, 121
  depression,
    major, 117, 121, 118
    psychotic, 119, 121
  dreaming, 119
  eating disorders, 121, 22, 23
  ecstasy, 124
  emotional disorders, 117
    general considerations, 121
  falling out, 124
  gallstones, 132
  hallucinations, 118-120
  headaches,
    cluster, 135, 27
    migraine, 135-6, 25-6, 149
    muscle tension, 132
    sinus, 132
    tension, 132
  heart attacks, 129
  hidden memory, 11, 13, 15-20,
    142-143,149-164,
  hydrocephalus, 132
  imagery, 115, 129, 114
  intensive care unit, 129
  insanity, 118
  irritable bowel syndrome, 134
  jet lag, 133

kidney stones, 131
kriyas, 125, 121
Kundilini, 123, 121
low back pain, 144
major depression, 117, 121
massage, 115
memory, hidden, 11, 13, 15-20,
  142-3, 149-164
menstrual,
  bleeding, excessive, 137
  distress, 137, 136
migraine, 135-6, 25-26, 149-164
night terrors, children's 121
nightmares, 119, 121
pain, 139, 127
  from a blow, 143, 121
  secondary, 141
phobias, 118, 121
physical therapy, 146
physioemotional reactions, 32
pregnancy, 133
premenstrual distress, 136, 137
psychiatric disorders, 117-121
  general considerations, 120
psychogenic shock, 131, 127
psychotic depression, 119, 121
rebirthing, 115
recovery
  from surgery, 130
  from trauma, 130, 131
Rolfing, 116
scheduling treatments, 112
schizophrenia, 118
secondary pain, 141
siddhas, 125
sinus headaches, 132
shock, 131, 27
spastic colon, 134, 16
stemming from a blow, 143
stones, gall, kidney, 132, 110
surgery, support of, 130
swollen,
  joints, 131
  leg, 32
  tissue, 127
tension headaches, 132
terrors, children's night, 121
tinnitus, 133
vertigo, 133

SHEN THERAPY PROTOCOLS, page xiv

SHEN treatment planning, 111-114
Shock, 131

Shorthand, SHEN, 165-166
Siddhas, 125
Site specificity, 11
Somatic affect, 6, 29, 47
  effects of repression, 7, 29
  reaction to, 7, 29
  site specific, 11
Somatoform disorders, 6
Specificity, anatomic, 11
Specifics, 127
Splinting reflex, 8
Sprains, 131
Sternomastoids, 87
Stone, Randolph, v
Stones,
  gall, 132
  kidney, 132
Stress, 3
  regional, 3, 10, 11, 42
Stressors, individual, 3
Subtle energies, v
Suggestability, 14, 22, 28
Surgery, 130
Swollen
  joints, 131
  leg, 32
  tissue, 127

T

Tables
  of emotion regions, 12
  language and emotions, 12
Temperature measurements from
  field effects, 58-60
Temperature rise during SHEN, 32
Therapeutic Touch, v
Thoughts,
  and emotion, 47-50
  confused, 50
  location of, 47
  rational, 49
Tinnitus, 133
Tissue, swollen, 127
Transducers, 57
Transformer action, 71
Transverse flows, 93
Treatment planning, 111-114

TREATMENT PROTOCOLS, page xiv

Triple flows, 88

V

Vertigo, 133

Vibrations, field, 66-67
Visceral brain, 47
Vortex, 67
Vortices, 67

W

Will, effort of, 77
Wind, rotary, 64

X

Xiphoid process, 87

NOTES

NOTES